GERONTOLOGIC NURSING

═══════ SECOND EDITION ═══════

Mary Ann Christ, RN, EdD, GNP
Dean
School of Nursing
University of Mississippi
Jackson

Faith J. Hohloch, RN, EdD
Professor Emeritus of Nursing
Medical University of South Carolina
Charleston

Springhouse Corporation
Springhouse, Pennsylvania

Staff

Executive Director, Editorial
Stanley Loeb

Director of Trade and Textbooks
Minnie B. Rose, RN, BSN, MEd

Art Director
John Hubbard

Clinical Consultant
Maryann Foley, RN, BSN

Editors
David Moreau, Kathy Goldberg

Copy Editor
Pamela Wingrod

Designers
Stephanie Peters (associate art director),
Jacalyn Facciolo

Typography
David Kosten (director), Diane Paluba (manager), Elizabeth Bergman, Joyce Rossi Biletz, Phyllis Marron, Robin Mayer, Valerie L. Rosenberger

Manufacturing
Deborah Meiris (manager), T.A. Landis, Anna Brindisi

©1993 by Springhouse Corporation, 1111 Bethlehem Pike, P.O. Box 908, Springhouse, PA 19477-0908. All rights reserved. Reproduction in whole or part by any means whatsoever without written permission of the publisher is prohibited by law. Authorization to photocopy items for internal or personal use, or the internal or personal use of specific clients, is granted by Springhouse Corporation for users registered with the Copyright Clearance Center (CCC) Transactional Reporting Service, provided that the base fee of $00.00 per copy plus $.75 per page is paid directly to CCC, 27 Congress St., Salem, MA 01970. For those organizations that have been granted a license by CCC, a separate system of payment has been arranged. The fee code for users of the Transactional Reporting Service is: 0874344883/93 $00.00 + $.75.

Printed in the United States of America.

SNGN-021092

Library of Congress Cataloging-in-Publication Data

Christ, Mary Ann.
  Gerontologic nursing/Mary Ann Christ, Faith J. Hohloch.—2nd ed.
    p. cm. — (Springhouse notes)
  Includes bibliographical references and index.
    1. Geriatric nursing. I. Hohloch, Faith J. II. Title. III. Series.
    [DNLM: 1. Geriatric Nursing—outlines. WY 18 C5544g]
RC954.C48   1993
610.73'65—dc20
DNLM/DLC   92-2320
ISBN 0-87434-488-3   CIP

Contents

Advisory Board and Reviewer

How to Use Springhouse Notes

Springhouse Notes is a multi-volume study guide series developed especially for nursing students. Each volume provides essential course material in an outline format, enabling the student to review the information efficiently.

Special features recur throughout the book to make the information accessible and easy to remember. *Learning objectives* begin each chapter, encouraging the student to evaluate knowledge before and after study. Next, within the outlined text, *key points* are highlighted in shaded blocks to facilitate a quick review of critical information. Key points may include cardinal signs and symptoms, current theories, important steps in a nursing procedure, critical assessment findings, crucial nursing interventions, or successful therapies and treatments. *Points to remember* summarize each chapter's major themes. *Study questions* then offer another opportunity to review material and assess knowledge gained before moving on to new information. Difficult, frequently used, or sometimes misunderstood terms (indicated by small capital letters in the outline) are gathered at the end of each chapter and defined in the *glossary*, Appendix A; answers to the study questions appear in Appendix B.

The Springhouse Notes volumes are designed as learning tools, not as primary information sources. When read conscientiously as a supplement to class attendance and textbook reading, Springhouse Notes can enhance understanding and help improve test scores and final grades.

CHAPTER 1

Demographics of Older Adults

Learning objectives

Check off the following items once you've mastered them:

☐ State what percentage of the U.S. population will be age 65 or older in the year 2030.

☐ Identify two factors that explain the large growth of the population age 65 or older.

☐ State the approximate percentage of older adults who live in institutions.

☐ Name the four most common chronic diseases in older adults.

☐ Identify the three most common causes of death in older adults.

I. Population statistics

A. Definitions
   1. An OLDER ADULT is an adult age 65 or older
   2. A YOUNG-OLD ADULT is an adult age 60 to 79
   3. An OLD-OLD ADULT is an adult age 80 to 99

B. General information
   1. In 1990, older adults accounted for 12.5% of the U.S. population
      a. The total population of older adults was 31 million
      b. This represents an increase of 5.3 million (21%) since 1980
   2. Since 1900, the older adult population has tripled as a percentage of the total population
      a. The greatest increase occurred in the population aged 65 to 74, which is eight times larger than it was in 1900
      b. The population aged 75 to 84 is 13 times larger than it was in 1900
      c. The population aged 85 and above is 24 times larger than it was in 1900
   3. In 1989, the net increase in the older adult population was 610,000 persons
      a. 2.2 million persons reached age 65
      b. 1.5 million persons age 65 or older died
   4. Between ages 65 and 69, women outnumber men by a ratio of 120 to 100; over age 85, women outnumber men by a ratio of 258 to 100

C. Projected growth of the older adult population
   1. Growth of the older adult population will peak in 2030
      a. The most rapid increase will occur from 2005 to 2030 as the baby-boom generation reaches age 65
      b. The growth rate will slow during the 1990s because of the lower birth rate during the Great Depression
   2. By 2000, older adults will make up 13% of the U.S. population
   3. By 2030, they will make up 21.8% of the U.S. population
   4. By 2030, the older adult population will be 2.5 times larger than it was in 1980
   5. By 2030, the population age 55 or older will be the only age group to experience significant growth

D. Factors contributing to the increased older adult population
   1. Mortality has declined
      a. A decrease in the rate of accidents and disease has resulted in fewer premature deaths
      b. Causes of this decrease include improved nutrition and sanitation, social improvements, disease prevention, and the health promotion and wellness movement
   2. Fertility has decreased

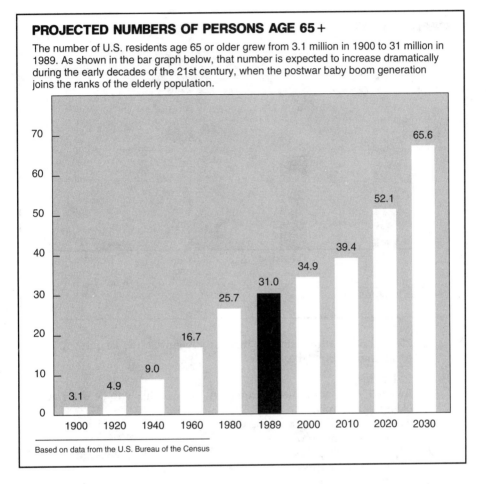

PROJECTED NUMBERS OF PERSONS AGE 65+

The number of U.S. residents age 65 or older grew from 3.1 million in 1900 to 31 million in 1989. As shown in the bar graph below, that number is expected to increase dramatically during the early decades of the 21st century, when the postwar baby boom generation joins the ranks of the elderly population.

Based on data from the U.S. Bureau of the Census

E. Life expectancy
   1. A child born in 1988 has a life expectancy of 74.9 years
   2. In 1988, a man age 65 had an average life expectancy of 79.8 years and a woman age 65 had an average life expectancy of 83.6 years

II. Racial and ethnic composition, marital status, and geographic distribution of older adults

A. Racial and ethnic composition
   1. In 1989, 90% of older adults were white
   2. 8% were black
   3. 3% were Hispanic

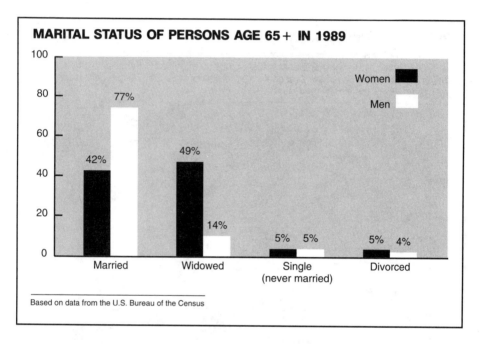

MARITAL STATUS OF PERSONS AGE 65+ IN 1989

Women ■
Men □

Married: Women 42%, Men 77%
Widowed: Women 49%, Men 14%
Single (never married): Women 5%, Men 5%
Divorced: Women 5%, Men 4%

Based on data from the U.S. Bureau of the Census

4. 2% had other ethnic origins, including Asian, Pacific Islander, Eskimo, Aleut, and Native American

B. Marital status
1. In 1989, older adult men were nearly twice as likely to be married as older adult women
2. 49% of older adult women were widows; widows outnumbered widowers by five to one
3. 4% of older adults had been divorced; the number of divorced older adults was four times higher than it was 20 years earlier

C. Geographic distribution
1. In 1989, 52% of older adults lived in nine states: California, New York, Florida, Illinois, Ohio, Pennsylvania, Texas, Michigan, and New Jersey
2. Older adults constituted 13.9% or more of the total population in 11 states: Florida, Arkansas, Rhode Island, Iowa, Pennsylvania, South Dakota, North Dakota, Missouri, West Virginia, Nebraska, and Oregon
3. Between 1980 and 1989, 10 states had more than 10% growth in the older adult population: Alaska, Nevada, Hawaii, Arizona, New Mexico, South Carolina, Utah, Florida, North Carolina, and Delaware
4. In 1989, approximately 74% of older adults lived in metropolitan areas

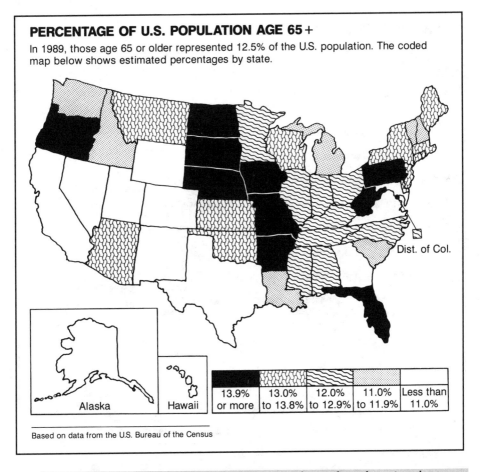

PERCENTAGE OF U.S. POPULATION AGE 65+

In 1989, those age 65 or older represented 12.5% of the U.S. population. The coded map below shows estimated percentages by state.

13.9% or more	13.0% to 13.8%	12.0% to 12.9%	11.0% to 11.9%	Less than 11.0%

Based on data from the U.S. Bureau of the Census

5. Older adults are less likely to change residence than those in other age groups
   a. Between 1980 and 1985, 16% of older adults moved
   b. The majority moved to another location in the same state
   c. Of those moving to a different state, 35% moved to a southern or western state

III. Economic status

A. Median income
   1. In 1989, the median income of older adults was $13,107 for men and $7,655 for women
   2. Families headed by an older adult had a median income of $23,179
      a. Whites had a median income of $23,817

PERCENT DISTRIBUTION BY INCOME

In 1989, older adults in the United States headed about 10.7 million family households (median annual income, $23,179) and 9.4 million nonfamily households (median annual income, $9,638).

Family households with head age 65 +

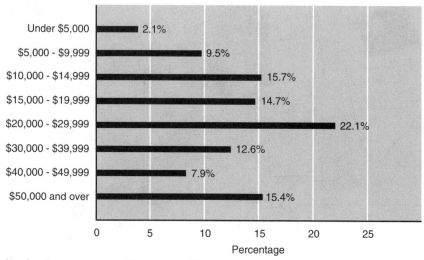

Nonfamily households with head age 65 +

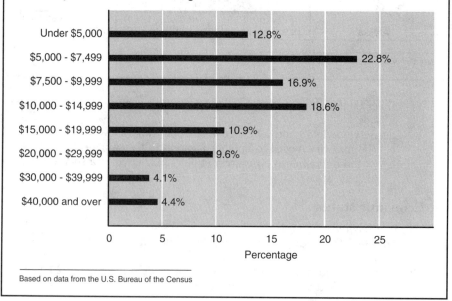

Based on data from the U.S. Bureau of the Census

      b. Blacks had a median income of $15,766

      c. 12% of families (one of every nine) had a median income below $10,000

      d. 36% of families had a median income of $30,000 or more

  3. Older adults who lived alone or in nonfamily households had a median income of $9,638

      a. 35.6% had an income of $7,500 or less

      b. 12.8% had an income of $5,000 or less

      c. 29% had an income of $15,000 or more

      d. Whites had a median income of $10,086

      e. Blacks had a median income of $6,035

B. Sources of income

  1. In 1988, Social Security accounted for 39% of the total income of older adults

  2. Asset income (income from interest, dividends, rental properties) accounted for 25% of total income

  3. Earnings accounted for 17% of total income

  4. Public and private pensions accounted for 17% of total income

  5. Supplemental Security Income, veteran's pension, and other sources accounted for 3% of total income

C. Median net worth

  1. In 1984, the median NET WORTH of the older adult's household was $60,000; this exceeded the U.S. average of $32,700

  2. 16% of older adults had a net worth below $5,000

  3. 7% had a net worth above $250,000

D. Poverty rate

  1. In 1989, 3.4 million older adults had incomes below the poverty level; this resulted in a poverty rate of 11.4% (in comparison, the poverty rate for persons under age 65 was 10.2%)

  2. 8% of older adults were classified as near poor

  3. 19% were classified as poor or near poor

  4. 10% of white older adults were classified as poor

  5. 31% of black older adults were classified as poor

  6. 21% of Hispanic older adults were classified as poor

  7. 14% of older adult women and 8% of older adult men were classified as poor

  8. Southern states had the highest poverty rates

IV. Health status

A. Aging and health

  1. AGING is a normal, universal, progressive, irreversible process

      a. Aging affects cells, organ systems, and body functions

      b. The rate of aging varies from one person to the next

      c. Factors affecting aging include genetic background, environment, activity pattern, and nutritional status

  2. The young-old population is relatively healthy and active; most persons in this age group function independently

  3. The old-old population experiences the impact of aging most directly, with chronic health problems exacerbating functional impairments

  4. Most older adults living in the community go out daily, manage their own care, and experience no illness requiring bed rest

  5. Most older adults rate their own health as good to excellent compared with others their age

      a. In 1988, about 29% assessed their health as fair or poor (in comparison, about 7% of persons under age 65 assessed their health as fair or poor)

      b. Nearly half of black older adults assessed their health as fair to poor

      c. Less than one-third of white older adults assessed their health as fair to poor

      d. Little difference in self-assessment of health status exists between the sexes at any age

B. Impact of chronic health problems and functional impairments

  1. Nearly one-fourth of older adults cannot manage self-care independently; about 10% receive help

  2. Activity limitation is the major consequence of chronic and acute health problems

      a. In 1988, older adults averaged 31 restricted days per year

      b. 14 of 31 (45%) restricted days were spent in bed

  3. In 1985, 5% of older adults lived in institutions, such as nursing homes or extended care facilities; most nursing home residents are age 85 or older, female, white, and widowed

  4. One in four older adults will spend some time in a nursing home

C. Chronic conditions affecting health

  1. Chronic illness is a major health problem in older adults

      a. Nearly 80% of older adults have at least one chronic health problem

      b. Many have multiple chronic health problems

  2. The physical health problems of older adults are wide ranging; common problems include arthritis, hypertension, hearing impairments, heart conditions, cataracts, sinusitis, orthopedic impairments, vision impairments, diabetes, tinnitus, and varicose veins

  3. Women have higher rates of all chronic health problems except hearing disorders

  4. The poor have the highest rate of all chronic health problems listed above

  5. Mental health problems in older adults include alcoholism, Alzheimer's disease and other dementias, and depression

D. Leading causes of death
  1. Among older adults, the 10 leading causes of death are heart disease; cancer; cerebrovascular disease; influenza and pneumonia; arteriosclerosis; diabetes mellitus; accidents; bronchitis, emphysema and asthma; cirrhosis of the liver; and nephritis and nephrosis
  2. Among older adult men, the 10 leading causes of death are heart disease; cancer; cerebrovascular disease; influenza and pneumonia; bronchitis, emphysema, and asthma; accidents; arteriosclerosis; diabetes mellitus; cirrhosis of the liver; and suicide
  3. Among older adult women, the 10 leading causes of death are heart disease; cancer; cerebrovascular disease; influenza and pneumonia; arteriosclerosis; diabetes mellitus; accidents; bronchitis, emphysema, and asthma; cirrhosis of the liver; and nephritis and nephrosis

V. Frail health and old-old adults

A. Demographics of the old-old population
  1. The fastest growing segment of the older adult population is over age 75
     a. Of noninstitutionalized adults age 75 to 84, about one-fourth need help with daily activities
     b. Of noninstitutionalized adults age 85 and older, nearly one-half need help with daily activities
     c. Those over age 75 who require help are called the *frail elderly*
  2. 22% of nursing home residents are over age 85

B. Characteristics of the frail elderly
  1. The frail elderly typically have a poor mental and physical health status
  2. They have a low income and socioeconomic status
  3. They are predominantly female
  4. Many live in isolation
  5. Compared with other older adults, the frail elderly have more and longer hospital stays, spend more money on health care and drugs, visit the physician more frequently, and occupy more nursing home beds than hospital beds

C. Factors contributing to frail health
  1. Some factors (for example, sex, ethnic group, and age) cannot be changed
  2. The cause of some factors, such as Alzheimer's disease, remains unknown
  3. Such factors as diet and exercise reflect life-style

D. Nursing considerations for the frail elderly
  1. This population is the most dependent and the most vulnerable to physical and mental impairment

2. They may need basic support to meet food, clothing, shelter, personal, medical, and financial needs
3. They may also need help with activities of daily living (ADLs)
   a. Physical ADLs include toileting, feeding, dressing, ambulating, and bathing
   b. INSTRUMENTAL ADLs include telephoning, shopping, preparing meals, cleaning house, doing laundry, obtaining transportation, taking medication, and managing finances
4. Needs of older adults who do not live in institutions are met through personal, family, and community resources: day care, neighborhood support groups, nursing centers or clinics, telephone support networks, foster families, and alternative residential care
5. Old-old persons in frail health usually are sicker than younger persons
6. The nurse's role includes assessing and assisting the old-old adult and taking preventive measures with the younger adult to promote health
   a. The nurse assesses the old-old adult's FUNCTIONAL ABILITY, assisting the patient and family to obtain needed resources or institutional placement when necessary
   b. The nurse works with the younger adult to change life-style to promote health and anticipate health consequences of life-style factors in later life

Points to remember

Aging is a universal shared experience.

Since 1900, the older adult population has tripled as a percentage of the total population.

Most young-old adults are independent, active citizens who can meet their own needs and lead satisfying lives.

Most old-old adults experience chronic health problems that exacerbate functional impairments.

Adults over age 75 constitue the most rapidly growing segment of the population.

Chronic illness usually has a major impact on adults age 85 and older.

Glossary

The following terms are defined in Appendix A, page 194.

aging	older adult
functional ability	old-old adult
instrumental ADLs	young-old adult
net worth	

Study questions

To evaluate your understanding of this chapter, answer the following questions in the space provided; then compare your responses with the correct answers in Appendix B, page 201.

1. Which two factors affect the age distribution of the population? _____

   _____

   _____

2. Which states had more than a 10% growth in the older adult population between 1980 and 1989? _____

   _____

3. Older adults derive income from which sources?_____

   _____

   _____

4. How do most older adults rate their health compared to others their age?

   _____

   _____

5. What are the two leading causes of death in older adults? _____

   _____

   _____

6. What is the fastest growing segment of the older adult population? _____

   _____

   _____

CHAPTER 2

Theories of Aging

Learning objectives

Check off the following items once you've mastered them:

☐ Name the three distinguishing characteristics of theories of aging.

☐ State one difference between genetic and nongenetic biological theories of aging.

☐ Describe how memory changes with age.

☐ Explain the difference between the disengagement theory and the activity theory.

I. General information

A. No universally accepted definition or theory of aging exists

B. Aging is a normal lifelong process that begins at conception
   1. GERIATRICS is the study of the diseases of aging
   2. GERONTOLOGY is the study of all aspects and problems of aging, including physiologic, pathologic, psychological, economic, and sociologic

C. Theories of aging must have three characteristics
   1. They must describe aging as universal in all members of a species
   2. They must describe aging as progressive over the life span
   3. They must describe aging as debilitative, leading to degenerative changes and failure of systems (however, not all systems may fail simultaneously)

D. All theories and concepts of aging are interrelated

E. Theories of aging may support or refute one another

F. Biological, psychological, and sociologic theories of aging exist

G. Several theorists have described the developmental tasks of aging (see Chapter 3, II)

II. Biological theories

A. Biological theories of aging attempt to explain physical aging changes

B. They define biological aging in two ways
   1. Aging is an involuntary process eventually leading to cumulative change, resulting in changes in cells, tissues, and fluids
   2. Aging involves structural alterations resulting from interaction with the environment, leading to degenerative changes

C. Biological theories may be intrinsic or extrinsic
   1. Intrinsic theories maintain that age-related changes arise from internal predetermined causes
   2. Extrinsic theories maintain that aging results from environmental factors that produce changes in the body
   3. Genetic theories are intrinsic
      a. Such theories posit the existence of a *biological clock*, an internal genetic control that determines the aging process (similar to a set time to live that winds down gradually)
         (1) The rate of aging differs from system to system within an organism
         (2) Some individual cells live longer than the organism
      b. Genetic theories maintain that each species has a characteristic life span

          (1) The maximum life span is species-specific (for example, 28 years for cats and 20 years for dogs)

          (2) The maximum life span for human beings is 115 years

      c. Most genetic theories include the concept of SOMATIC MUTATION, which refers to a failure or an error in the replication of deoxyribonucleic acid

      d. The *programmed aging theory* holds that cells divide in vitro about 50 times and no more (Hayflick limit)

  4. Nongenetic theories are extrinsic

      a. The FREE RADICAL theory holds that an increase in unstable free radicals from environmental pollutants alters the biological system, leading to changes in chromosomes, pigment, and collagen with aging

      b. The *cross-link theory* holds that collagen molecules and chemicals alter tissue function, leading to tissue stiffness and rigidity with aging

      c. The *immunologic theory* holds that lymphoid tissue changes cause an imbalance in T cells

          (1) This leads to a decrease in cellular immune function

          (2) The result is autoantibody production and immune deficiencies

  5. Physiologic theories are both intrinsic and extrinsic

      a. The *stress adaptation theory* holds that stress response activation causes accumulated damage; stressors may be internal (physical or psychological) or external (social or environmental)

      b. The *wear-and-tear theory* holds that after repeated injury or use, body structures and functions wear out from stress

III. Psychological theories

A. Psychological theories of aging attempt to explain aging changes in cognitive functions (intelligence, memory, learning, and problem solving)

B. They posit the following age-related changes in cognitive functions

  1. *Intelligence* is affected by age somewhat

      a. FLUID INTELLIGENCE decreases slightly

      b. CRYSTALLIZED INTELLIGENCE does not decrease

      c. In very old age, both crystallized and fluid intelligence decline

      d. Intelligence decreases about 5 years before death

  2. *Memory* undergoes various age-related changes

      a. PRIMARY MEMORY (information held in temporary storage for active processing) remains intact; however, storage capacity for primary memory is limited

      b. SECONDARY MEMORY (information that is held in storage and must be retrieved) declines with age

          (1) Storage for secondary memory is permanent and unlimited in capacity

          (2) Ability to retrieve information from storage decreases with age

   (3) An example of an age-related decrease in secondary memory
       is reduced ability to perform tasks requiring organizational
       and elaborative processes (for instance, list learning or
       orienting tasks)
  c. SHORT-TERM MEMORY (which encompasses components of both
     primary and secondary memory) declines with age from difficulty
     retrieving information from secondary memory
  d. LONG-TERM MEMORY (also called remote memory) undergoes
     minimal change
  e. Decreased ability to acquire new material and retrieve information
     from storage is a major age-related memory change
  f. Age-related memory decreases can be minimized by using
     organization and elaboration techniques, repetition and practice,
     self-regulation of pace, and individual learning methods
  g. Changes in memory are affected by environment
3. *Learning and problem solving* also are affected by age
  a. Learning is influenced by lack of stimulating changes and the
     tendency for older adults to learn only useful information
  b. An age-related increase in arousal levels before and after learning
     situations may increase errors
  c. The ability to solve complex problems declines
  d. The capacity to retain meaningful information remains unaltered
  e. Learning and problem solving are affected by the environment

IV. Sociologic theories

A. Sociologic theories of aging attempt to explain aging changes that affect
   socialization and life satisfaction

B. No single theoretical framework on the social aspects of aging exists

C. Sociologic theories hold that age is not a good predictor of social behavior

D. Sociologic theories, derived from social psychology, are based on the
   following assumptions
   1. Stratification by age is necessary for the organization of society
   2. Social structures determine an individual's rights and responsibilities
   3. Aging cannot be explained fully using only biological theories
   4. Social expectations occur over the course of a lifetime; some remain
      constant while others change
   5. New social expectations lead to changes in identity (for instance,
      retirement or a sick role)

E. Sociologic theories include the social exchange theory, disengagement
   theory, activity theory, and continuity theory
   1. The *social exchange* theory holds that social behavior involves doing
      what is valued and rewarded by society

    a. Older adults have decreased resources and increased dependency; consequently, they have less power and value and their contribution to society is reduced

    b. With advancing age comes a decrease in the number of roles available in society

    c. Roles change with age

       (1) The parental role is completed as children mature

       (2) The worker role disappears with retirement

    d. Old age may bring on new roles, such as volunteer, friend, grandparent, and widow or widower

    e. Proximity of other people is crucial to maintaining a social network

    f. Effects of forced changes in socialization patterns (for example, increased or decreased interaction with others) are unknown

    g. Friendships with peers help socialize an older adult to age-related norms

       (1) Such norms include those of retirement, grandparenthood, and widowhood

       (2) Socialization is an age-related process

       (3) Few elderly models or mentors exist to serve as examples

    h. Age-related expectations change with time and culture

       (1) Each COHORT and generation develop specific expectations (for instance, women's roles have changed over time)

       (2) Social and historical events (such as the Great Depression and world wars) affect expectations

    i. For most older persons, a spouse's death brings only a minimal change in physical or psychosocial adaptation

    j. The need for intimacy continues until death

       (1) Some older adults transfer needs fulfillment to friends after a spouse dies; women find this easier to do than men

       (2) Men commonly meet the need for companionship by remarrying

2. The *disengagement theory* was proposed by Elaine Cumming and William Henry in the 1950s

    a. It holds that aging brings progressive social disengagement that is mutual and acceptable to both the individual and society

    b. Other theorists suggest that the degree of disengagement varies with individual personality and life activity pattern and that the level of activity (social involvement) is a lifelong pattern that remains constant

    c. Studies show that changes in health, energy, income, and roles affect the older adult's disengagement and activity pattern

    d. Disengagement theory reflects the observation that some older adults have decreased participation in society; it does not hold true for most older adults

    e. This theory does not consider social structure variables, such as the economy or social organizations

      f. It also does not take into account the diversity of outlook and life-style among older adults

  3. The *activity theory* was developed by Frances Carp and others in 1966

      a. This theory proposes that successful aging depends on maintaining a high activity level and that life satisfaction is related to involvement in life

      b. Quality and meaningfulness of an activity are more important than the number of social activities a person participates in

      c. Studies show that when activities in one area decrease, activities in another area increase

      d. The impact of a decrease or other change in activities on development of social isolation is unknown

      e. The impact of other aging or health changes (such as diminished sensory perception) is unknown

      f. Like the disengagement theory, the activity theory does not take into account the diversity of outlook and life-style among older adults

  4. The *continuity theory* assumes the stability of individual patterns or orientation over time

      a. This theory asserts that the individual self remains essentially the same despite life changes

      b. It focuses more on personality and individual behavior over time

      c. It does not take into account major societal changes that alter individual expectations and behaviors, such as changes in women's roles

      d. The continuity theory assumes that an activity-pattern preference is maintained over the course of a lifetime

V. Nursing implications of theories of aging

A. No one theory explains aging

B. The various theories help direct areas to be assessed

C. Theories suggest areas in which older adults experience changes, how they make major life changes, and how they may experience stress or crises

D. Theories also provide guidelines for assessing an older adult's adjustment to aging and can help identify health promotion needs

E. Theories allow consistent nursing approaches

F. Theories offer rationales for specific interventions

Points to remember

No universally accepted biological, psychological, or sociologic theory of aging exists.

Various theories are interrelated and may support or refute one another.

Short-term memory decreases with age because older adults have difficulty retrieving information from secondary memory.

Cognitive functions, socialization, life satisfaction, and environmental interaction undergo age-related changes.

Older adults collectively are characterized by diversity, not similarity.

Glossary

The following terms are defined in Appendix A, page 194.

cohort	long-term memory
crystallized intelligence	primary memory
fluid intelligence	secondary memory
free radical	short-term memory
geriatrics	somatic mutation
gerontology	

Study questions

To evaluate your understanding of this chapter, answer the following questions in the space provided; then compare your responses with the correct answers in Appendix B, page 201.

1. Theories of aging must include which three characteristics? _____

    _____

    _____

2. How do intrinsic biological theories of aging differ from extrinsic biological theories of aging? _____

    _____

3. Psychological theories of aging attempt to explain which changes? _____

    _____

    _____

4. What does the activity theory of aging propose? _____

    _____

CHAPTER 3

Age-Related Transitions

Learning objectives

Check off the following items once you've mastered them:

☐ Name five basic human needs that people of all ages share.

☐ Define ageism.

☐ Identify four role changes that occur with aging.

☐ Name one major factor causing loneliness.

I. Basic human needs

A. Basic concepts
   1. Every human being has needs
   2. How a person meets needs affects growth and development
   3. Age-related changes interact with basic human needs
   4. Abraham Maslow proposed a framework, or hierarchy, for prioritizing human needs
      a. Physical needs come first, followed by security, love, trust, self-esteem, and self-actualization
      b. A person has concerns at every level of the needs hierarchy
      c. With age, concerns about the ability to meet physical needs increase
   5. Various other needs also exist
      a. *Identity* refers to having one's own name, family connections, uniqueness in life history, and body image; changes in stature and appearance may affect self-image and identity
      b. *Rootedness* denotes having a place in time and space
      c. *Relatedness* refers to having someone to relate to, such as a confidant
      d. *Transcendence* denotes the quality of no longer being preoccupied with ordinary, mundane matters
      e. *Understanding* refers to the power to make experience intelligible
      f. *Usefulness* is a feeling of being needed and wanted
      g. *Recognition* denotes being viewed as a person of worth
      h. *Social involvement* refers to the need to interact with others

B. Nursing implications
   1. Acknowledge and address the basic human needs of the older adult patient when planning care
   2. Set realistic expectations based on these needs
   3. Teach the patient about age-related changes in the body and self-image and provide emotional support
   4. Assess the patient's adjustment to aging, including self-image, growth and self-actualization, integration of personality, autonomy, realistic perception of the self and world, and environmental mastery
   5. Establish intervention strategies to promote healthy adjustment to aging
      a. Maximize the patient's abilities and resources (for instance, encourage the patient to make decisions independently and to extend the social network)
      b. Promote adaptation to changing internal needs and external requirements (for example, assist with life-style adjustments and changes in income)
      c. Maintain or increase the patient's capacity for responding to personal needs and environmental challenges, such as by helping the patient acquire skills to manage chronic disease

   d. Ensure that nurses become involved in designing programs and developing policies that address major variables affecting successful aging (such as poverty, AGEISM, and social isolation)

II. Developmental task theories

A. Basic concepts
   1. Developmental task theories describe specific life stages and tasks associated with each stage
   2. Developmental tasks are steps to be accomplished in a process that a person experiences during growth and maturity
   3. Developmental task theorists describe what they believe is expected at each life stage; many developmental task theories exist
   4. Developmental task theories may be interrelated and may support or refute one another as well as other theories of aging
   5. Developmental task theories hold that age is a major factor in determining life stage
   6. They also hold that behavior appropriate at one stage may be inappropriate at another

B. Erik Erikson's theory
   1. This theory describes eight developmental stages and specific tasks, based on Freudian theory, that occur throughout the life span
      a. Stage I (infancy): trust vs. mistrust
      b. Stage II (toddler): autonomy vs. shame and doubt
      c. Stage III (preschool): initiative vs. guilt
      d. Stage IV (school age): industry vs. inferiority
      e. Stage V (adolescence): identity vs. identity diffusion
      f. Stage VI (adulthood): intimacy vs. isolation
      g. Stage VII (middle adulthood): generativity vs. stagnation
      h. Stage VIII (old age): integrity vs. despair
   2. Each developmental stage is characterized by specific tasks
   3. Tasks to be met involve biological, psychological, and cultural aspects of aging
   4. Task resolution involves various behaviors
      a. Adjusting to old age
      b. Believing that one's life is meaningful and important
      c. Integrating one's life to prepare for death
      d. Recognizing that the past cannot be changed
   5. Successful resolution of stage VIII promotes ego integration; unsuccessful completion results in despair
   6. Successful aging and completion of developmental tasks lead to wisdom

C. Vivian Clayton's theory
   1. Clayton investigated Erikson's concept of integrity and its ego attribute, wisdom

2. Clayton's theory views old age as a psychosocial crisis that disturbs old ego structures, and defines wisdom as the ability to adjust one's perceptions of reality. This is done by:
   a. Seeing new meaning in past experiences
   b. Reexamining the meaning of life

D. Robert Peck's theory
   1. This theory describes tasks related to development of integrity
   2. It holds that successful task resolution requires a person to develop the ability to reach a higher level of awareness, redefine the self, and move beyond self-centeredness
   3. It proposes that the person may be unsuccessful, unable to let go of a previous role or to create new meaning
   4. This theory proposes the following tasks:
      a. Ego differentiation vs. work-role preoccupation
      b. Body transcendence vs. body preoccupation
      c. Ego transcendence vs. ego preoccupation

E. Bernice Neugarten's theory
   1. This theory describes increased *interiority* (a growing interest in inner development) as a task of the older adult
   2. It proposes that a person's inward focus increases with age
   3. It holds that inward focus may result from an internal need for self-actualization or from an age-related change in environment that causes withdrawal (such as retirement)
   4. Neugarten was the first to develop the concept of the young-old age group (age 55 to 74) and old-old (age 75 or older) age group; others have used her concept with different age groupings
   5. She postulated that a continuity of behavioral patterns develops over time and that stability outweighs change
   6. According to her theory, aging women move from relatively passive modes to active modes; aging men move from relatively active to passive modes
   7. Her theory refers to a social time clock, a set of age-related norms for movement through the phases of adulthood (for example, the "right" time to retire)
   8. It holds that the older adult experiences discomfort when engaging in roles or functions at a socially defined inappropriate time
   9. It also proposes that old age has fewer socially defined norms

F. Lawrence Kohlberg's theory
   1. This theory describes six stages of moral development and proposes that the crises of adult life are moral dilemmas that lead to moral development
   2. It describes the last stage of moral development as the universal ethic principle orientation (development of a personal ethical value system)
   3. Morality is defined by and within a person's cultural values

    4. Questions about personal and social value lead a person to redefine the self
    5. Most moral dilemmas of old age relate to interpersonal concerns
    6. Moral problems of old age include:
      a. Problems with family, such as giving and taking advice, caregiving and living arrangements, and financial resources
      b. Problems with societal or legal expectations
      c. Problems related to work or retirement
      d. Problems related to personal freedom
      e. Problems with friends and neighbors
        (1) Involvement in others' affairs
        (2) Involvement in others' safety or welfare

G. Robert Havighurst's theory
    1. This theory describes developmental tasks of adulthood that result in satisfactory growth
    2. It defines tasks as bio-socio-psychological; that is, tasks require the person to adjust to physical changes (such as decline in strength), psychological changes (such as loss of a spouse), and social changes (such as different living arrangements)
    3. It defines successful aging as flexible adaptation to new roles within social customs
    4. It identifies six tasks of later life
      a. Adjusting to declining physical strength and health
      b. Adjusting to retirement and reduced income
      c. Adjusting to changes in the spouse's health
      d. Establishing an explicit affiliation with one's age group
      e. Adopting and adapting social roles in a flexible way
      f. Establishing satisfactory physical living arrangements

H. Robert Butler's theory
    1. This theory proposes that reminiscence and life review are critical to an older adult's growth and the development of wisdom and serenity
    2. It proposes that life review is an adaptive function of aging and dying
    3. It views reflection on regrets or disappointments as a catalyst for deeper self-awareness
    4. Butler coined the term *ageism* to describe discrimination against older adults

III. Developmental task accomplishment

A. Basic concepts
    1. Achievement of developmental tasks promotes happiness and successful adjustment
    2. Achievement helps the older adult view aging as a positive or PEAK EXPERIENCE

3. Major tasks relate to achieving and maintaining integrity vs. despair, according to Erikson and Peck
   a. Ego differentiation vs. role preoccupation (establish valued activities and new roles and let go of the work role)
   b. Body transcendence vs. body preoccupation (focus on comfort, activities, and enjoyment rather than on pain and losses)
   c. Ego transcendence vs. ego preoccupation (focus on how valuable life has been and on one's legacy rather than death; develop a self-transcending philosophy; accept death; teach others about dying)
4. Havighurst also proposed that developmental tasks also relate to social, physical, and psychological losses experienced by the older adult
   a. Developmental tasks focus on various behaviors
      (1) Reorganizing functions and expectations
      (2) Adjusting spending patterns to retirement income
      (3) Changing functions in the marital relationship during retirement
      (4) Adjusting living arrangements to meet safety, independence, and physical function requirements
      (5) Adjusting to changes in body function and ability to perform activities
   b. Maladjustment occurs if an individual fails to accept and adapt to changing physical abilities and health
   c. Developmental tasks stress various needs
      (1) The need to associate with other older adults
      (2) The need to change the perception of old age
      (3) The need to become politically involved in activities aimed at improving the health and social services available to older adults
   d. Developmental tasks lead to various goals
      (1) Reappraising personal worth in light of loss of the work role
      (2) Finding a source of self-worth beyond the work role identity
      (3) Using leisure time to establish alternative meaningful activities
   e. Developmental tasks stress the need to face the reality of death and to ensure children's welfare
   f. Developmental tasks require active effort to gain closure of life and involve the drive for self-perpetuation and the need to leave a legacy
   g. Developmental tasks lead to a period of critical self-assessment and reevaluation of life successes and failures
   h. Developmental tasks stress the need to maintain self-acceptance, self-esteem, and positive self-concept while adapting to diminished health, social support, and resources

B. Factors associated with task accomplishment
   1. The older adult must cope with multiple losses successfully
   2. The older adult must relinquish power and capacity (be willing to give up or give in)

3. The older adult must develop compensatory behaviors; adjust to change; and develop new skills, friends, and roles

C. Nursing implications
   1. Incorporate assessment and interventions for developmental tasks into nursing care
   2. Serve as an advocate with families, health professionals, and society to promote aging as a positive experience
   3. Recognize and reinforce positive compensatory behaviors

IV. Transitions and role changes

A. Basic concepts
   1. Aging is associated with many role changes and transitions
      a. Some roles (such as spouse, friend, occupation) are lost
      b. Role adjustment (such as adjusting to retirement or a sick role) is required
      c. New roles (such as widow or volunteer) arise
      d. Relocation may bring role changes and transitions
   2. Changes in marital roles take place
      a. Division of labor may change after retirement
      b. Social relations change if the spouse dies
      c. Household management also changes
      d. One spouse may become the primary caregiver if the other becomes ill
      e. Spouses may need to renegotiate household roles and leisure and social activities
   3. Retirement brings a major role change
      a. It alters the way a person manages time and daily activities
      b. The retiree must adapt to a nonworker role
      c. Others also must adjust (for example, the spouse may view retirement as a threat to territoriality and authority)
      d. Retirement alters identity, power, status, and friendships
      e. The retiree may need to find new relationships and activities; women usually develop new friendships more easily than men
      f. Retirement is seen as the beginning of old age
      g. Income, health, and the desire to retire affect satisfactory adjustment to retirement
      h. Those with more income and education seem better prepared for retirement
      i. Some organizations offer preretirement counseling; some employees may be able to cut back on work hours gradually to retire in stages
      j. Adjusting to retirement may be easier if a person begins postretirement activities before retiring
   4. Older adults also undergo other role changes
      a. The *parent role* may change

(1) As an older adult becomes more dependent, reversal of roles in the parent-child relationship occurs

(2) Increased dependency causes loss of power, status, and decision making

b. The *grandparent role* usually begins

(1) Most people take on this role by age 70

(2) This role usually is a supportive, companionship role

c. The *independent adult role* erodes gradually

(1) This change stems mostly from increased dependency

(2) Stereotypes about the elderly contribute to erosion of the independent adult role; for example, health professionals may view older adults as unreliable historians and thus discount their self-reports

d. A *sick role* may arise from multiple interactive health problems resulting from chronic disease and limited power to negotiate care

5. Relocation may cause changes in roles, health, income, and type of housing

B. Factors associated with role adjustment

1. Age, sex, culture, beliefs, attitudes, income, health, and past experiences affect a person's adjustment to role changes

2. Although change may be a single event, the effect is *interactive* with all areas of life

C. Nursing implications

1. Provide guidance for the older adult regarding attitudes and expectations, identifying new sources of satisfaction and new roles and activities

2. Support preretirement discussion of role changes by the patient and spouse

3. Encourage preretirement planning and counseling about income, living arrangements, social and leisure activities, and health care

4. Assist with retirement planning; this is a key health promotion activity because successful adjustment is crucial to healthy aging

V. Attitudes and beliefs

A. Basic concepts

1. Attitudes are learned through one's culture

2. American cultural attitudes are diverse yet they share many similarities

a. They value performance, productivity, appearance, self-reliance, independence, and individuality

b. They are youth-oriented

c. They derive from the Puritan work ethic, which stressed work, productivity, and contribution

d. They view human beings as mechanistic

      e. They view the body and mind as separate entities

      f. Society devalues older adults, viewing them as obsolete and expendable; this makes older adults feel worthless

  3. Beliefs affect attitudes and feelings

      a. Beliefs vary with experience, culture, and religious values

      b. Many people fear changes associated with aging

  4. Older adults are the most stereotyped age group

      a. Negative stereotyping of older adults appears in literature, in jokes, and on television; this perpetuates ageism

      b. A poor parent-child relationship or negative childhood experiences may contribute to a negative attitude toward aging

  5. Social attitudes are changing

      a. Society is adjusting its attitudes about aging as the older adult population increases and older adults take on new roles

      b. More emphasis now is placed on being a worthwhile individual and on viewing the developmental process as unilateral and old age as the culmination of life

      c. A more humanistic approach is emerging, with more attention paid to obligations to others and to self development

      d. Changes in viewpoint have led to the recognition of human beings as open and evolving (organismic model)

      e. More positive attitudes about old age now exist in many younger people, better-educated people, and people who have had contact with healthy older adults

      f. New roles and an increasing sense of self-worth are emerging for older adults

B. Effects of stereotypes about old age

  1. Stereotypical attitudes and beliefs result in myths (such as the myth that all old people are alike, poor, sick, depressed, destined to become senile, or incapable of change)

  2. Stereotypical attitudes and beliefs can affect health care workers and health care delivery

      a. They may affect all aspects of care planning and implementation (for example, they may cause a delay in answering an older adult's call bell)

      b. They may affect a person's choice of career and job selection

      c. Stereotypes also influence salaries; for instance, nurses working in nursing homes typically make less money than those working in other health care facilities

      d. Stereotypes also affect policy and program development

C. Nursing implications

  1. Examine personal attitudes and beliefs about aging

  2. Sensitize others to stereotypical attitudes and beliefs about older adults and aging and teach about their impact on the care of older adults

VI. Religion

A. Basic concepts
   1. Religion may be a source of support for an older adult
   2. The older adult typically continues the religious pattern developed in earlier adulthood
   3. Religion can help define self-worth and identity
   4. Cultural emphasis on religion varies
   5. Religion gives meaning to life and helps integrate life experiences
   6. Only 3% of older adults have no religious affiliation
   7. Rituals and prayers offer hope
   8. The older adult may seek religious support from church personnel to help deal with emotional problems
   9. Churches provide social activities amd crisis help
   10. Church supportive services involve no cost, waiting lines, or records that may create a stigma

B. Factors associated with religious practice
   1. Immobility or transportation problems may curtail the older adult's attendance at religious services
   2. Strict adherence to religious practice may necessitate special diets for some older adults
   3. After the death of a loved one, some older adults may become disenchanted with or more involved in religion
   4. Older adults with limited income may withdraw from religion because they do not have the money they perceive as necessary to contribute to a religious organization

C. Nursing implications
   1. Support the patient's religious beliefs and practices
   2. Find out what the patient wants
      a. Do not assume the patient desires religious consultation or participation in services
      b. Do not assume religion is the patient's source of support
   3. Be aware that spiritual well-being is as important as physical and psychological well-being

VII. Losses

A. Basic concepts
   1. Aging is associated with major physical, psychological, and sociologic losses
   2. Older adults have a reduced ability to adapt to and compensate for stressors
   3. They experience a decreased sense of control and increased dependency from such factors as loss of the decision-making role, impact of negative cultural attitudes, crime victimization, mass media portrayal of elderly persons as helpless, and status and role changes

4. They may suffer cumulative loss of internal and external resources, relationships, and roles (such as loss of loved ones, income, and decent housing and transportation)
5. Cumulative losses combined with multiple or chronic diseases and limitations increase the older adult's vulnerability
6. Cumulative losses also may deplete coping resources
7. All losses necessitate grieving
    a. The stages of grief must be completed so that grief can be resolved
    b. Stages of grief include shock, denial, anger, guilt, depression, understanding, and acceptance
    c. Duration of each stage varies
    d. Not all individuals go through all stages
    e. Stages may not proceed sequentially
    f. Grieving may last 1 to 2 years
    g. Unresolved grief leads to prolonged sadness and depression, which may be translated into physical complaints
    h. Anticipatory grieving, in which one begins grieving when confronted with impending loss, promotes movement through grief
8. Positive aging allows the older adult to overcome losses
9. Losses and such contributing factors as loneliness, depression, and fear of death are interrelated and may exacerbate one another

B. Factors associated with loss
    1. *Loneliness* may result from multiple losses, which create deficits in intimacy and interpersonal relationships
        a. The older adult needs caring, personal contact, and confidants in other age groups
        b. Loneliness may be associated with decreased survival and complaints of physical symptoms and sleep disturbances
        c. Sensory deprivation is associated with an increased risk of loneliness
        d. The older adult needs a satisfying relationship with a frequent contact to prevent loneliness
        e. Not all loneliness can be avoided
        f. Death of a spouse is a major cause of loneliness
        g. Retirement, poor health, and inactivity contribute to loneliness
    2. *Depression* is more likely in the older adult
        a. The frequency and intensity of depression increase with age
        b. Changes in neurotransmitters, multiple losses, and decreased internal and external resources make depression more likely in the older adult
        c. Depression may occur in early stages of dementia
        d. Depression is the most common psychiatric problem among older adults

      e. Risk factors for depression include a recent major loss, feelings of rejection by or isolation from family or friends, feelings of hopelessness, absence of an identifiable role in life, and loss of a sex partner or sexual function

      f. Depression is the most common psychological consequence of disability

      g. Depression increases the suicide risk

         (1) The suicide rate of older adult men is seven times that of older adult women

         (2) A person may seek death actively through overt or covert suicide

         (3) Older adults account for about 25% of suicides

         (4) White men are at greatest risk for suicide

         (5) Risk factors for suicide include alcoholism, bereavement (especially within 1 year after a loss), loss of health, living alone, and children marrying and moving away

         (6) Suicide among older adults *rarely* is an impulsive act

         (7) Most suicide attempts are not gestures or threats

      h. Depression may be associated with complaints of physical symptoms and sleep disturbance

   3. *Fear of death* may involve such concerns as the afterlife, judgment, and separation from loved ones

      a. Death is the natural outcome of living and cannot be controlled; denial of death prevents one from valuing life

      b. Preparation for death can be a positive experience; it is a major developmental task

      c. Older adults commonly think and talk about death; most other people avoid the topic

      d. Older adults have less fear of death than younger people (the greatest fears of older adults are dependency, pain, and loss of function and control)

      e. The United States has a DEATH-DENYING culture

C. Nursing implications

   1. Recognize loneliness and intervene to counteract it and increase the older adult's socialization

      a. Resources include family support, community programs, pet therapy, and crisis intervention

      b. If the patient lacks support systems, establish a network of neighbors, friends, church, and telephone contacts

   2. Support the patient in working through grief

   3. Determine if the patient has considered suicide or has a plan for doing so; keep in mind that someone with a well-planned method (especially a lethal one) is at higher risk for suicide

   4. Refer the patient with unresolved grief, depression, or thoughts of suicide for counseling

5. Promote the patient's expression of feelings and loss
6. Support the patient to mobilize compensatory behaviors and encourage active participation in life
7. Recognize the interrelationship of age-related changes and loss of resources
8. Suggest that the patient find a substitute for lost companionship (such as a pet or new social connections)
9. Encourage participation in group activities
10. Involve the patient's family in care plans and activities
11. Encourage reminiscence and life review as a way to integrate life experiences and resolve losses
    a. Reminiscence refers to thinking about and reflecting on the past
    b. Life review is the structured reminiscence of life accomplishments using life stages and the recognition that one has lived the best way one could
    c. This process involves action-oriented intervention
    d. It also involves allowing patients to talk about themselves
    e. The nurse can promote and enhance this process by helping to trigger memories and listening with empathy
    f. Patients may need help in summarizing their lives and integrating meaning into them
    g. Life review involves active recall of unresolved conflicts, accomplishments, and failures
    h. An individual or group approach to reminiscence and life review may be used
    i. The process incorporates traumatic events and normative crises (crises associated with normal life events, such as the death of a sibling)
    j. Methods include written or taped autobiographies, pilgrimages, reunions, genealogies, scrap books, and albums

Points to remember

Multiple losses and changes in internal and external resources decrease the older adult's ability to meet basic human needs independently.

Healthy aging experiences give older adults an opportunity to transcend losses.

Negative stereotypes of aging and older adults perpetuate ageism.

Depression is the most common psychiatric problem among older adults.

Twenty-five percent of suicides occur among older adults.

Glossary

The following terms are defined in Appendix A, page 194.

ageism

death-denying

ego integrity

peak experience

Study questions

To evaluate your understanding of this chapter, answer the following questions in the space provided; then compare your responses with the correct answers in Appendix B, pages 201 and 202.

1. To determine the older adult's adjustment to aging, the nurse should assess which factors? _____

   _____

2. Robert Peck described which developmental tasks? _____

   _____

3. What are three factors associated with role adjustment in the older adult?

   _____

   _____

4. How do stereotypical attitudes affect the health care profession? _____

   _____

   _____

5. Which nursing interventions related to religion are appropriate for the older adult? _____

   _____

CHAPTER 4

Age-Related Physical Changes

Learning objectives

Check off the following items once you've mastered them:

☐ Describe how age-related changes in the cardio-vascular system affect cardiac output, blood pressure, and heart rate.

☐ Identify four age-related changes in the gastrointestinal system that affect the mouth.

☐ Name age-related changes that affect renal function.

☐ Identify two types of anatomic brain lesions that are associated with aging.

☐ Describe age-related changes in vision and hearing.

☐ State how age-related changes in estrogen and insulin production affect the body.

I. Changes in posture, appearance, and body composition

A. Progressive increase in the severity and extent of age-related changes affecting all cells, organs, and systems

B. Posture
1. Typically, aging causes a person to stoop forward, with the head tilted backward and the knees, hips, and elbows flexed
2. Postural changes stem from various causes
   a. Body proportions are altered
      (1) Shoulder width decreases
      (2) The chest, pelvic, and abdominal areas increase in diameter
   b. Bones lose calcium and cartilage and muscles undergo changes, contributing to structural changes
   c. The trunk shortens as intervertebral distances narrow and vertebrae become thinner
   d. The center of gravity moves from the hips to the upper torso; this affects balance

C. Appearance
1. Decreases in skin elasticity, height, subcutaneous fat, and bone mass cause marked changes in appearance
2. The result may be an overall bony appearance, with sunken eyes, prominent forehead, and accentuation of elongated ears

D. Body composition
1. By age 75, body fat (adipose tissue) increases by 16% overall
   a. The proportion of body fat to lean mass increases
   b. Lean body mass declines by about 15% over the life span
   c. The arms and legs lose body fat while the abdomen and hips gain body fat
2. By age 75, body water decreases by 8%
   a. The amount of intracellular water decreases (from a change in cellular mass)
   b. The amount of extracellular water remains the same
   c. Total body water decreases
3. Weight changes reflect changes in body composition
   a. Men over age 55 lose weight gradually (20 pounds or more)
   b. Women typically gain weight until age 60, when weight decreases gradually

II. Structural and functional changes in the integumentary system

A. Skin
1. Cellular turnover declines from slow cell reproduction in the epidermis and dermis
   a. Skin cell replacement drops by about 50%
   b. Skin healing decreases significantly

      c. Pigmentation undergoes change, with spotty patterns appearing in sun-exposed areas
  2. Blood supply to the skin decreases
      a. The greatest decrease occurs in the arms and legs
      b. Vascular fragility increases, contributing to development of SENILE PURPURA (more common in women)
  3. Subcutaneous fat is lost
      a. The greatest loss occurs in the arms and legs
      b. Men lose more subcutaneous fat than women
      c. Subcutaneous fat loss contributes to decreased cold tolerance
  4. The skin becomes thinner
      a. Skin elasticity decreases
      b. Collagen bundles become larger and stiffer
      c. Skin wrinkling and sagging result
      d. The epidermis becomes thin and fragile
  5. Decreases in cellular turnover, blood supply, subcutaneous fat, and skin thickness cause reduced wound healing and increase the risk of decubitus ulcer formation

B. Sweat glands
  1. Sweat glands decline in size, number, and function
  2. This causes dry skin, decreased perspiration, and reduced ability to regulate body temperature

C. Hair
  1. Hair growth decreases
  2. Melanin production declines
      a. Graying of the hair results
      b. Genetic factors determine onset of graying
  3. The pattern of hair growth changes
      a. In men, hair growth on the scalp decreases while hair growth on the ears and eyebrows increases; beard growth remains unchanged
      b. In women, axillary and pubic hair become sparser after menopause
      c. Facial hair growth is common in Caucasian women

D. Nails
  1. Nail growth and nail strength decrease
  2. Longitudinal nail ridges become more numerous and prominent

III. Structural and functional changes in the respiratory system

A. Chest structures
  1. Skeletal muscles, connective tissue, and smooth muscle become more rigid
      a. Inspiratory and expiratory muscle strength declines, causing reductions in ventilation and vital capacity
      b. The intercostal and scalene accessory muscles and diaphragm are used more for expiration than they were used previously

   2. Anteroposterior chest diameter increases
   3. The posterior thoracic curve increases, leading to kyphosis
   4. The cough mechanism is less effective because of inadequate force (which results from anatomic chest changes and reduced muscle strength)
   5. The rib cage becomes more rigid
   6. Costal cartilage becomes calcified

B. Lungs
   1. The greatest change occurs after age 70
   2. Respiratory fluids decrease by about 30%
     a. This decrease affects mucous membranes and respiratory tract secretions, thereby drying the airways
     b. It also increases the risk of mucus obstruction and infection
   3. Changes in elastin and collagen components of lung tissue and pulmonary blood vessels lead to reduced diffusion activity
     a. Tensile strength and flexibility decrease
     b. Recoil during expiration decreases
     c. Thickening of the capillary basement membrane and reduction in the number of vessels lead to decreased diffusion
   4. Increased apical ventilation and decreased basilar ventilation cause poor ventilation of lung bases
   5. Functional capacity drops by about 50%
     a. This results in dyspnea with exertion or stress
     b. No functional changes occur at rest
   6. Inspiratory reserve volume decreases
   7. Expiratory reserve volume increases from residual air in the lung bases at the end of expiration
   8. Oxyhemoglobin saturation decreases by about 5%
   9. Blood pH and partial pressures of arterial oxygen and carbon dioxide remain unchanged
  10. Total lung capacity and tidal volume remain unchanged
  11. The lungs become rigid
  12. Alveoli decrease in number and size

IV. Structural and functional changes in the cardiovascular system

A. Heart
   1. Cardiac enlargement occurs in some older adults; however, this is not a proven age-related change
   2. The left ventricle becomes about 25% thicker
   3. Myocardial elasticity decreases; rigidity increases
   4. Valves thicken and become rigid
   5. The endocardium thickens from fibrosis and sclerosis
   6. Fat infiltration occurs; connective tissue decreases
   7. Lipofuscin (aging pigment) appears in cardiac cells

8. Ability of the heart rate to increase with stress declines (however, the resting heart rate remains unchanged)
9. Stroke volume and cardiac output decrease by about 1% each year between ages 19 and 86
10. Tachycardia is tolerated poorly
    a. The heart needs more time to resume a normal rate
    b. Exercise, emotions, and fever may cause sinus tachycardia, which may lead to cardiac arrhythmias or heart failure
11. Blood flow to all organs decreases; the brain and coronary arteries receive a larger blood volume than other organs and structures
12. Coronary artery blood flow decreases by about 35% between ages 20 and 60
13. Recovery of myocardial contractility is delayed
14. Myocardial irritability increases, possibly causing extra systoles
15. Electrocardiogram (ECG) shows specific changes
    a. P-R, QRS, and Q-T intervals increase
    b. QRS complex amplitude decreases
    c. The QRS axis shifts to the left

B. Blood vessels
    1. Arterial elasticity declines, causing increased peripheral resistance
    2. Calcium deposits in the arterial media increase, leading to fibrosis and sclerosis
    3. Vessel stretch decreases about 50% by age 80
    4. Superficial vessels become more prominent
    5. The aorta and carotid artery become tortuous
    6. The capillary basement membrane thickens
    7. Valves in the veins become less efficient; varicose veins or stasis ulcers may develop
    8. Veins become dilated, stretched, and tortuous
    9. Systolic blood pressure and heart work increase in response to greater peripheral resistance; diastolic blood pressure rises slightly
    10. Altered blood flow distribution and increased peripheral resistance cause major physiologic changes, such as arteriosclerosis, hypertension, and diminished tissue perfusion

V. Structural and functional changes in the gastrointestinal system

A. Teeth
    1. Tooth enamel thins; teeth become brittle
    2. Tooth loss is not a normal age-related change

B. Mouth
    1. Saliva production decreases, causing dry mouth and a diminished sense of taste
    2. Taste buds decrease in number
    3. Biting force declines

    4. The gag reflex decreases

C. Esophagus
1. Decreased peristaltic activity and relaxation of the lower esophageal sphincter cause delayed emptying and an increased risk of aspiration
2. Increased frequency of hiatal hernia may result from age-related changes

D. Stomach
1. Fat tissue accumulates and smooth muscle thins, resulting in delayed gastric emptying and difficulty in managing large food quantities
2. Pepsin and hydrochloric acid secretion decrease
   a. This causes minimal functional change
   b. Absorption of calcium and vitamins B_1 and B_2 diminishes; however, the amount absorbed is adequate
3. Production of intrinsic factor decreases; however, the decrease is not sufficient to cause pernicious anemia

E. Small intestine
1. Nutrient absorption may decline
2. No significant functional changes occur

F. Large intestine
1. The musculature weakens
2. Peristalsis decreases
3. Nerve sensation diminishes
4. The external sphincter reflex decreases
5. Constipation may occur from age-related changes, inadequate diet, and reduced exercise patterns
6. Intestinal cell replacement takes twice as long
7. Diverticulosis of the sigmoid colon occurs in one third of persons over age 60

G. Liver
1. Liver size decreases after age 70
2. Hepatic enzyme concentration decreases
3. Enzyme response to external stimuli declines
4. Enzymes of hepatic microsomes active in oxidation and reduction reactions decline markedly; this affects drug metabolism and detoxification
5. Ability to synthesize protein from the liver decreases; however, functional capacity of the liver remains normal

H. Gallbladder
1. Emptying becomes more difficult
2. Bile decreases in amount and becomes thicker
3. Gallstones develop in approximately 40% of persons by age 80; however, the incidence is not linked to aging
4. The cholesterol content of bile increases

I. Pancreas
1. The enzymes trypsin, amylase, and lipase decrease in volume and concentration
   a. This reduction may be associated with poor tolerance of high-fat meals and poor absorption of fat-soluble vitamins
   b. Enzyme concentrations remain sufficient to maintain digestive function
2. Bicarbonate secretion remains unchanged
3. Insulin release diminishes (for details, see "Structural and functional changes in the endocrine system," page 44)

VI. Structural and functional changes in the genitourinary system

A. Kidney
1. The number of nephron units decreases; glomeruli and tubules undergo progressive changes
2. Kidney size decreases from reduced renal tissue growth
3. The amount of extracellular fluid increases and cell mass decreases
4. The GLOMERULAR FILTRATION RATE (GFR) decreases
   a. This decrease stems from a 53% reduction in renal blood flow (from decreased cardiac output), which also reduces renal efficiency (50% of residual function is sufficient for renal function)
   b. The decline in GFR begins around age 40; by age 90, GFR is about 50% lower than at age 20
   c. Decreased GFR causes reduced renal clearance of drugs
5. Glucose reabsorption from filtrate decreases by 43.5%
6. By age 70, the blood urea nitrogen (BUN) level increases by 21%
7. Urine-concentrating ability diminishes (especially at night) from changes in tubular function
8. Reduced muscle mass leads to decreased production of CREATININE
   a. Consequently, the creatinine clearance test (a urine and blood test) should be corrected for age
   b. The creatinine clearance test is the best index of renal function in older adults
9. Because of reduced muscle mass, the serum creatinine level (measured from a blood test) does not rise, despite decreased renal function
10. The BUN level increases up to 30 mg/dl
11. Sodium-conserving ability decreases
12. Acid-base disturbances take longer to correct
13. Chronic diseases of older adults, such as atherosclerosis, further reduce renal function

B. Bladder
1. Bladder capacity decreases by half
   a. Urinary frequency and nocturia increase

      b. Some older adults void every 2 hours during the day and once at night (they may need to void 30 minutes after going to bed because a recumbent position increases renal function)

  2. Bladder shape changes from pearlike to funnel-like

  3. Emptying becomes more difficult from weakening of the bladder and perineal muscles and changes in the sensation of the voiding urge

      a. This causes retention of large volumes of urine

      b. In men, increased frequency or dribbling may result from a weakened bladder or an enlarged prostate gland

      c. In women, stress incontinence may result from weakening of the pelvic diaphragm, which is caused by childbirth

C. Female reproductive organs

  1. Ovaries become smaller and fibrotic

  2. Estrogen production diminishes with menopause

  3. Breast tissue decreases

  4. The uterus and cervix undergo various changes

      a. They become smaller

      b. Mucus secretion stops

      c. Muscle weakening may lead to uterine prolapse

  5. The vagina also undergoes various changes

      a. The vaginal canal becomes narrower and shorter

      b. The epithelial lining atrophies

      c. Vaginal secretions become more alkaline

      d. Vaginal elasticity decreases

      e. The risk of atrophic vaginitis increases

  6. Libido remains unchanged

D. Male reproductive organs

  1. The testicles become smaller

  2. Testosterone production decreases

  3. The sperm count falls

  4. Seminal fluid becomes less viscous

  5. The prostate gland enlarges (at very advanced ages, it may atrophy)

  6. Libido remains unchanged

VII. Structural and functional changes in the neurologic system

A. Brain

  1. Atrophy occurs, reducing brain size by as much as 7%

  2. The gyri become atrophic; the sulci and ventricles become dilated

  3. Cerebral blood flow and oxygen use decrease

  4. Neurons are lost

      a. Neurons do not regenerate; loss is permanent and inevitable

      b. Neuron loss is most pronounced in the cerebral cortex, which loses about 20% of its neurons

      c. Lipofuscin (aging pigment) appears in cytoplasm

      d. Protein synthesis decreases

      e. The hypothalamus becomes less effective in regulating heat
         production and heat loss

      f. Senile plaques and neurofibrillatory tangles (anatomic lesions
         associated with aging) develop; plaques and tangles occur in older
         adults *with and without* dementia

B. Peripheral nerves

  1. Deep tendon reflexes decrease

  2. Peripheral nerve conduction diminishes by about 15%

     a. The number of dendrites in nerves decreases

     b. Changes in synapses occur, slowing nerve impulse conduction

     c. This causes a slow reaction time

     d. Lesions form on axons

  3. Function of the autonomic and sympathetic nervous systems decreases

C. Neurotransmitters

  1. Monoamine oxidase and serotonin levels increase and norepinephrine
     levels decrease; this may contribute to depression in older adults

  2. The dopamine level decreases (the decrease is more pronounced in
     patients with Parkinson's disease)

VIII. Structural and functional changes in the endocrine system

A. Pituitary gland

  1. The vascular network decreases

  2. Connective tissue increases

  3. No change occurs in concentration and secretion of
     adrenocorticotropic hormone, thyroid-stimulating hormone, growth
     hormone, and luteinizing hormone

  4. Secretion of follicle-stimulating hormone increases in postmenopausal
     women but remains unchanged in men

B. Thyroid gland

  1. Such structural changes as fibrosis and follicular distention occur;
     however, no functional changes result

  2. The plasma thyroxine level remains unchanged

  3. The plasma triiodothyronine level decreases 25% to 40%

  4. The metabolic rate slows

C. Parathyroid gland

  1. Some structural changes occur; however, atrophy and degeneration
     remain minimal

  2. Experts do not know if aging causes a decrease in parathyroid
     hormone secretion

D. Pancreas

  1. Insulin release and peripheral sensitivity decrease

  2. Glucose tolerance declines with age

3. Experts do not know if aging affects glucagon

E. Adrenal glands
   1. Secretion of glucocorticoids decreases
      a. The cortisol secretion rate drops about 25%
      b. The urinary excretion rate of glucocorticoids drops about 25%
      c. These decreases cause no adverse effects
   2. The blood level and urinary excretion of aldosterone decrease by about 50%
   3. Urinary excretion of the 17-ketosteroids decreases by about 50%

F. Gonads
   1. Estrogen production ceases with menopause
      a. This causes atrophy of the ovaries, uterus, and vagina
      b. It also ends reproductive capacity
   2. Progesterone production by the ovaries, testes, and adrenal cortex declines after the reproductive period ends
   3. The metabolic clearance rate and production rate of testosterone decline (the ovary continues to secrete testosterone after menopause)

IX. Structural and functional changes in the musculoskeletal system

A. Bone
   1. Bone loss starts at approximately age 40
   2. Diet, hormonal changes, and physical activity affect the rate of bone loss
   3. The bone reabsorption rate exceeds the rate of new bone formation
   4. Trabecular bone loss exceeds cortical bone loss
   5. Bone loss is universal; it affects about 25% of women and about 12% of men (for details, see Chapter 5, Section XVIII)
   6. Bone loss predisposes older adults to fractures

B. Muscles
   1. Muscle cells are lost and not replaced
      a. Remaining muscle cells atrophy (the degree of muscle wasting can be observed on the dorsum of the hand)
      b. Total muscle mass decreases
   2. The proportion of muscle weight to body weight decreases
   3. The size of the motor unit decreases; muscle strength declines 10% to 20%
   4. Prolonged impulse conduction time leads to slowing of impulses along the motor unit
   5. Muscle fatigability increases from changes in enzyme activity

C. Joints
   1. Changes start to develop between ages 20 and 30 as cartilage erosion begins

2. Synovial membranes become friable; synovial fluid thickens
3. Intervertebral disks undergo bone loss
   a. Decreased water content in intervertebral disks contributes to a decrease in height
   b. Degenerative changes cause the nucleus pulposus to lose turgor and become friable
   c. Osteophytes form on the vertebral column, causing osteoarthritic changes; cervical osteoarthritis develops in about 25% of persons over age 50

X. Structural and functional changes in the sensory system

A. Vision
   1. Multiple structural changes result in PRESBYOPIA
   2. The lens becomes discolored, opaque, and rigid, leading to cataract formation
   3. Changes in the lens and vitreous humor cause decreased visual acuity
   4. Decreased depth of the anterior chamber and reduced aqueous humor reabsorption may cause glaucoma
   5. The pupil becomes smaller, reducing the amount of light striking the retina
   6. The eye's ability to adapt to darkness decreases
   7. ARCUS SENILIS appears around the iris

B. Hearing
   1. Multiple structural changes result in PRESBYCUSIS (progressive, bilaterally symmetrical perceptive hearing loss); presbycusis impairs the ability to understand speech
   2. Loss of high-frequency hearing usually occurs before loss of middle- or low-frequency hearing
   3. Tone discrimination decreases

C. Gustation (taste) and olfaction (smell)
   1. Taste buds decrease in number; remaining taste buds atrophy
   2. Sensitivity for all tastes decreases
   3. Experts do not know if olfaction also declines

XI. Structural and functional changes in the immune system

A. Thymus
   1. This gland is essential for production of T lymphocytes (T cells), which control the body's ability to respond to ANTIGENS and provide protection against tumor formation and foreign cells
   2. Beginning at puberty, the thymus undergoes involution (progressive degeneration)
      a. At age 50, only 5% to 10% of the thymus mass remains
      b. By age 60, no thymic hormones are produced
      c. The response to antigenic stimuli decreases

B. Other changes
   1. Natural antibodies decrease in number
   2. Autoantibodies increase, causing a greater risk of autoimmune disorders
   3. ANTIBODY response to antigens declines
   4. Cellular and humoral immunity diminish
   5. These changes reduce the chance of survival

XII. Changes in homeostasis and functional reserve

A. HOMEOSTASIS
   1. Physiologic, psychological, and social factors must be integrated to maintain homeostasis
   2. Age-related changes reduce the body's ability to maintain homeostasis
      a. With age, adaptive mechanisms may be taxed beyond their ability to respond; deterioration occurs unless stress is reduced and balance is restored
      b. Physiologic, mental, and behavioral responses to homeostatic stress become more erratic with age; more effort is needed to restore dynamic homeostasis

B. FUNCTIONAL RESERVE
   1. With age, functional reserve (body's ability to adapt to changes) in many systems decreases
   2. Stresses within one or more systems deplete the body's adaptive capacity
   3. Decreased functional reserve and depleted adaptive capacity increase vulnerability to additional stressors, including illness, psychological stress, and environmental changes

Points to remember

Age-related changes affect all cells, organs, and systems.

Body fat increases with age, whereas body water decreases.

Age-related integumentary system changes include decreased cellular turnover, reduced blood supply, loss of subcutaneous fat, and thinning of skin.

In the older adult, inspiratory reserve volume decreases and expiratory reserve volume increases.

Cardiac enlargement is not a proven age-related change.

Decreased functional reserve may leave the older adult vulnerable to additional stressors.

Glossary

The following terms are defined in Appendix A, page 194.

antibody	glomerular filtration rate
anitgen	homeostasis
arcus senilis	presbycusis
creatinine	presbyopia
functional reserve	senile purpura

Study questions

To evaluate your understanding of this chapter, answer the following questions in the space provided; then compare your responses with the correct answers in Appendix B, page 202.

1. By age 75, which changes in body fat and body water occur? ⎯⎯⎯⎯⎯⎯⎯

⎯⎯⎯⎯⎯⎯⎯⎯⎯⎯⎯⎯⎯⎯⎯⎯⎯⎯⎯⎯⎯⎯⎯⎯⎯⎯⎯⎯⎯⎯

⎯⎯⎯⎯⎯⎯⎯⎯⎯⎯⎯⎯⎯⎯⎯⎯⎯⎯⎯⎯⎯⎯⎯⎯⎯⎯⎯⎯⎯⎯

2. Which structural and functional changes in the skin result from aging?

⎯⎯⎯⎯⎯⎯⎯⎯⎯⎯⎯⎯⎯⎯⎯⎯⎯⎯⎯⎯⎯⎯⎯⎯⎯⎯⎯⎯⎯⎯

⎯⎯⎯⎯⎯⎯⎯⎯⎯⎯⎯⎯⎯⎯⎯⎯⎯⎯⎯⎯⎯⎯⎯⎯⎯⎯⎯⎯⎯⎯

3. How does aging affect pulmonary alveoli? ⎯⎯⎯⎯⎯⎯⎯⎯⎯⎯⎯⎯⎯

⎯⎯⎯⎯⎯⎯⎯⎯⎯⎯⎯⎯⎯⎯⎯⎯⎯⎯⎯⎯⎯⎯⎯⎯⎯⎯⎯⎯⎯⎯

4. Which ECG changes are associated with aging? ⎯⎯⎯⎯⎯⎯⎯⎯⎯⎯⎯

⎯⎯⎯⎯⎯⎯⎯⎯⎯⎯⎯⎯⎯⎯⎯⎯⎯⎯⎯⎯⎯⎯⎯⎯⎯⎯⎯⎯⎯⎯

5. What are the effects of age-related accumulation of fat tissue in the stomach?

⎯⎯⎯⎯⎯⎯⎯⎯⎯⎯⎯⎯⎯⎯⎯⎯⎯⎯⎯⎯⎯⎯⎯⎯⎯⎯⎯⎯⎯⎯

⎯⎯⎯⎯⎯⎯⎯⎯⎯⎯⎯⎯⎯⎯⎯⎯⎯⎯⎯⎯⎯⎯⎯⎯⎯⎯⎯⎯⎯⎯

6. At what age does the GFR start to decline? ⎯⎯⎯⎯⎯⎯⎯⎯⎯⎯⎯⎯

⎯⎯⎯⎯⎯⎯⎯⎯⎯⎯⎯⎯⎯⎯⎯⎯⎯⎯⎯⎯⎯⎯⎯⎯⎯⎯⎯⎯⎯⎯

7. How does aging affect neurotransmitters? ⎯⎯⎯⎯⎯⎯⎯⎯⎯⎯⎯⎯⎯

⎯⎯⎯⎯⎯⎯⎯⎯⎯⎯⎯⎯⎯⎯⎯⎯⎯⎯⎯⎯⎯⎯⎯⎯⎯⎯⎯⎯⎯⎯

8. How does aging affect glucose tolerance? ⎯⎯⎯⎯⎯⎯⎯⎯⎯⎯⎯⎯⎯

⎯⎯⎯⎯⎯⎯⎯⎯⎯⎯⎯⎯⎯⎯⎯⎯⎯⎯⎯⎯⎯⎯⎯⎯⎯⎯⎯⎯⎯⎯

9. Which changes in intervertebral disks contribute to decreased height in older adults? ⎯⎯⎯⎯⎯⎯⎯⎯⎯⎯⎯⎯⎯⎯⎯⎯⎯⎯⎯⎯⎯⎯⎯⎯

⎯⎯⎯⎯⎯⎯⎯⎯⎯⎯⎯⎯⎯⎯⎯⎯⎯⎯⎯⎯⎯⎯⎯⎯⎯⎯⎯⎯⎯⎯

CHAPTER 5

Age-Related Disorders

Learning objectives

Check off the following items once you've mastered them:

☐ Recognize that signs and symptoms of disorders in older adults may vary from those found in younger persons.

☐ Name the most common eye problem in older adults.

☐ Identify the most common cause of respiratory disability in older adults.

☐ Describe nursing interventions that help prevent decubitus ulcers.

☐ Identify abnormal laboratory or X-ray findings for older adults with common pathologic health problems.

I. Acute confusional states

A. General information
1. *Acute confusional state* refers to an irreversible disturbance in cognitive function
2. Some references (including the *Diagnostic and Statistical Manual of Mental Disorders*, third edition, revised [*DSM-III-R*]) prefer the term DELIRIUM for all confusional states
3. Previously, acute confusional states were termed *acute or reversible brain syndrome*
4. Acute confusional states may progress from disorientation to delirium
5. Such states have a variable onset
   a. They sometimes develop over a short period (hours to days)
   b. However, usually they evolve gradually over several months, such as when caused by systemic illness or metabolic imbalance (the brain of an older adult is more sensitive to body changes during illness than that of a younger person)
6. Acute confusional states range from quiet disorientation or reduced cooperation with care to agitated states with impaired attention, perception, memory, and thinking; hallucinations, illusions, or delusions also may occur
   a. The terms *hallucination, delusion*, and *illusion* should not be used interchangeably
   b. Hallucinations are auditory, visual, gustatory, olfactory, or tactile perceptions that arise without external stimuli
   c. Delusions are persistent false beliefs that are held firmly even though they are based on incorrect or illogical inferences
   d. Illusions are false or misinterpreted external sensory stimuli, usually visual or auditory in nature
7. Acute confusional states can result from infection, neurologic factors, cardiorespiratory factors, endocrine and metabolic conditions, electrolyte imbalances, nutritional factors, environmental factors, and other conditions
   a. Infections that can cause an acute confusional state include bronchopneumonia, local skin lesions, diverticular abscess, and bacterial endocarditis
   b. Neurologic factors include drugs with central nervous system (CNS) action, cerebral arteriosclerosis, stroke, brain tumor, subdural hematoma, and epilepsy
   c. Cardiorespiratory factors include myocardial infarction (MI), congestive heart failure (CHF), pulmonary emboli, respiratory failure, and acute hemorrhage
   d. Endocrine and metabolic conditions include hypothyroidism, hypoglycemia, hyperglycemia, hyperparathyroidism, and an elevated blood urea nitrogen (BUN) level

    e. Electrolyte imbalances that can cause an acute confusional state include dehydration, renal failure, and hypercalcemia

    f. Nutritional factors include cachexia and B_{12} or thiamine deficiency

    g. Environmental factors include decreased sensory input, sensory overload, and sudden isolation

    h. Other factors that can trigger an acute confusional state include anesthetic agents, surgical or accidental trauma, tissue anoxia, gangrene, and digitalis toxicity

  8. Acute confusional states increase psychological stress and may lead to further mental deterioration

  9. Older adults with DEMENTIA are especially vulnerable to acute confusional states

10. Sensory deprivation and an unfamiliar environment contribute to acute confusional states

11. If an acute confusional state is not treated promptly, permanent deterioration of cognitive function may result

12. Acute confusional states have a negative effect on both the patient's health and the nurse's ability to provide care (for example, they can impair communication and expose the patient or nurse to injury)

B. Assessment findings

  1. Signs and symptoms of acute confusional states may be subtle and may vary throughout the day

  2. The patient may be forgetful or disoriented

  3. Ability to shift focus or sustain attention is impaired

  4. Other signs and symptoms include memory loss, disordered speech, misinterpretation of reality, hallucinations, restlessness, a disturbed sleep-awake cycle, anxiety, and delusions of persecution

  5. Tachycardia, sweating, facial flushing, pupil dilation, and blood pressure elevation may accompany the acute confusional state

  6. Acute confusional states usually last less than 1 week

C. Nursing implications

  1. Keep in mind that nursing goals are to establish a meaningful environment; to help maintain body awareness; and to help the patient cope with confusion and any hallucinations, delusions, or illusions

  2. Place the patient near a window, if possible, to help differentiate between day and night

  3. Keep calendars and clocks in a location where the patient can see them easily

  4. Determine what is perceived from the patient's vantage point; illusions commonly result from a limited perspective of an unfamiliar environment

  5. Allow the patient to sit in a chair for short periods during the day to help improve the patient's perceptions of the environment

  6. Be aware that an acute confusional state may stem from sudden body changes, such as fever, pain, trauma, and acute onset of an illness

7. If the patient exhibits agitation or unsafe behavior, ask in a soft, calm voice what specific help the patient needs (for example, ask "Are you looking for the bathroom?")

8. Implement safety measures to protect the patient from pulling out tubes or falling

9. Help maintain body awareness by allowing the patient to explore and identify (under careful supervision) foreign objects, such as tubes or a colostomy

10. Reinforce the patient's identity by using life history events to focus on areas of competence and promote a sense of self-worth while minimizing factors contributing to confusion

11. Help the patient deal with any hallucinations, delusions, and illusions by verifying statements and identifying facts; describe reality in a slow, calm manner

12. Identify correctable factors that may trigger confusion after dark, such as fatigue, unmet toileting needs, increased noise, decreased light, sedatives and pain medications, and fewer staff members

13. Be aware that decreased sensory stimulation in an unfamiliar environment during the night may cause confusion in older adults with marginal cerebral reserve; this phenomenon, commonly called sundowning, is *not* an acute confusional state

D. Evaluation
   1. The patient's signs and symptoms are managed appropriately
   2. The patient avoids injury

II. Arterial insufficiency

A. General information
   1. Arterial insufficiency is an interference in arterial blood flow that results from narrowing or blockage of an artery
   2. The condition can be acute or chronic
      a. Acute arterial insufficiency has a sudden onset indicating complete arterial blockage, which can cause serious tissue ISCHEMIA
      b. Chronic arterial insufficiency develops gradually from plaque accumulation
   3. Arterial insufficiency may result from:
      a. Arterial embolism
      b. Arterial thrombosis
      c. ARTERIOSCLEROSIS OBLITERANS
      d. Vascular changes caused by diabetes mellitus
      e. Trauma
   4. Risk factors for arterial insufficiency include:
      a. Male sex with a history of hypertension and an inherited predisposition to cardiovascular or peripheral vascular disease
      b. Smoking
      c. Diabetes mellitus

  d. Hypercholesterolemia

  e. Obesity

  f. Stressful life-style

 5. In older adults, arteriosclerosis obliterans is the most frequent cause of arterial insufficiency resulting in ischemic lesions of the extremities

 6. Clinical manifestations and management of arteriosclerosis obliterans depend on the location and extent of the occlusive process

 7. The femoral, popliteal, and tibial arteries most commonly are involved in older adults; the aorta and iliac artery also may be involved

 8. In a patient with diabetes mellitus, arterial insufficiency is complicated by three major etiologic factors:

  a. Peripheral vascular changes

  b. Neuropathy

  c. Infection

 9. Diabetes mellitus accelerates the process leading to development of arteriosclerosis obliterans

 10. Factors that increase the risk for acute arterial insufficiency include:

  a. Invasive arterial procedures, such as arteriography

  b. Atrial fibrillation

  c. Vascular surgery

  d. Proximal aneurysm of the abdominal aorta or popliteal artery

  e. Arterial laceration, severance, or compression

B. Assessment findings

 1. Onset of pain may be sudden in acute arterial insufficiency or gradual in chronic arterial insufficiency

 2. Intermittent CLAUDICATION may accompany chronic arterial insufficiency; typically, this problem is relieved by rest

 3. Pulses in the affected extremity may be absent or weak

 4. Chronic arterial insufficiency may cause the following changes in legs and feet:

  a. Thin, dry, shiny skin

  b. Thickened nails

  c. Absence of hair

  d. Temperature variation between the left and right sides of the extremity

  e. Pallor on elevation

  f. Dependent erythema

  g. Atrophy with decreased limb size

 5. Ulcers may appear between the toes, at the tip of the toes, over phalangeal heads, on the heel, and over the lateral malleolus or pretibial area; in the diabetic patient, ulcers may arise on the metatarsal heads and on the side or sole of the foot

 6. Ulcers resulting from chronic arterial insufficiency have the following characteristics:

  a. Well-defined edges

     b. Black or necrotic tissue
     c. Deep base
     d. Pale color
     e. Absence of bleeding
  7. In acute arterial occlusion, the occlusion site is tender to the touch; other signs and symptoms include:
     a. Sudden burning or aching pain in an area distal to the occlusion
     b. Pain exacerbated by movement
     c. Numbness
     d. Pallor
     e. Cold to the touch
     f. Weakness
     g. PARESTHESIA
     h. Weak or absent pulse

C. Nursing implications
  1. Keep in mind that the nursing goal is to identify early signs and symptoms of acute or chronic arterial insufficiency to delay ischemic changes and relieve pain in affected extremities
  2. Know that for chronic arterial insufficiency, nursing interventions include:
     a. Encouraging the patient to engage in a progressive walking program to promote development of collateral circulation
     b. Advising the patient to take slow walks two or three times a day, using short steps, avoiding stairs and hills, and increasing the distance gradually
     c. Instructing the patient to stop walking if pain arises
     d. Ensuring that exercise is modified to prevent anginal pain (if the patient has a history of angina)
     e. Teaching the patient how to control such risk factors as obesity, smoking, diabetes, and hypercholesterolemia
     f. Administering analgesics or narcotics for pain relief, as ordered
     g. Teaching the patient the importance of meticulous daily foot care to prevent ischemic ulcers and infection
     h. Advising the patient to place lamb's wool between overlapping toes to separate them and prevent ulcers
     i. Cautioning the patient to avoid extreme hot and cold and warning the patient not to use heating pads, hot water bottles, and hot soaks to prevent thermal injury
     j. Instructing the patient to avoid constricting garments, such as girdles, garters, and tight hose or shoes, to prevent impaired circulation
  3. Know that for acute arterial insufficiency, treatment depends on the cause of occlusion and the patient's general health; nursing interventions may include:

      a. Protecting the affected limb by keeping it straight and at room temperature
      b. Administering anticoagulation therapy, if ordered
      c. Assessing pulses and motor and sensory responses frequently in the affected limb
      d. Checking for symmetry in limb size and shape

D. Evaluation
  1. The patient experiences relief of symptoms and improved arterial circulation
  2. The patient avoids ischemic changes

III. Cardiac arrhythmias

A. General information
  1. *Arrhythmia* refers to a disturbance in heart rate, rhythm, or both
  2. The disturbance may involve impulse formation, conduction, or both
  3. The incidence of cardiac arrhythmias increases with age
  4. Age-related changes in the heart (such as fibrosis, loss of muscle mass, increased collagen, calcification, and coronary artery occlusion) contribute to arrhythmias
  5. Factors that may trigger cardiac arrhythmias include:
      a. Myocardial ischemia
      b. Hypokalemia
      c. Systemic infection
      d. Blood loss
      e. Digitalis toxicity
  6. Arrhythmias are more serious in older adults because advanced age reduces tolerance for decreased cardiac output, which in turn may lead to syncope, falls, transient ischemic attacks, and possibly dementia
  7. Depending on the severity, an arrhythmia may precipitate angina, embolus or thrombus formation, MI, cardiovascular insufficiency, or death in older adults

B. Assessment findings
  1. Clinical features of arrhythmias result from compromised circulation and oxygen deficit
  2. Signs and symptoms of arrhythmias include:
      a. Changes in mentation, personality, and behavior
      b. Decreased blood pressure
      c. Chest pain
      d. Dizziness
      e. Dyspnea
      f. Tachypnea
      g. Pale, cool, clammy skin

3. Arrhythmias can cause myocardial ischemia with its attendant signs and symptoms, such as dyspnea, blood pressure fluctuation, and angina
4. In older adults, arrhythmias may precipitate CHF; signs and symptoms of CHF include dyspnea, fluid retention, and blood pressure changes
5. Electrocardiography (ECG) reveals specific arrhythmias and heart rhythm changes
6. Holter monitoring (tape-recorded ECG) commonly is used to diagnose paroxysmal arrhythmias that may be associated with symptoms and activities
7. The pulse may be rapid, slow, or irregular, depending on the specific arrhythmia

C. Nursing implications
1. Keep in mind that the nursing goal is to prevent, assess, and manage arrhythmia
2. Assess for signs of hypoperfusion (changes in mentation, hypotension, and diminished urine output) if the pulse is abnormally rapid, slow, or irregular
3. Stay alert for life-threatening arrhythmias by assessing frequently for level of consciousness, respirations, blood pressure, cardiac rhythm, and pulse; initiate cardiopulmonary resuscitation if a life-threatening arrhythmia arises
4. Expect to assist with treatment of underlying health problems that precipitate arrhythmias, such as infection and cardiac or pulmonary disorders
5. Expect to administer antiarrhythmic drugs, depending on the specific arrhythmia
6. Expect to eliminate substances that may trigger arrhythmias, including digitalis and other cardiac medications; encourage the patient to eliminate alcohol and cigarettes
7. Take measures to correct electrolyte imbalances, which may precipitate arrhythmias
8. If the patient is receiving digitalis, be aware of drugs (such as thiazide and loop diuretics) that may affect digitalis absorption
9. Carefully monitor patients receiving digitalis for signs and symptoms of digitalis toxicity:
   a. Anorexia
   b. Nausea
   c. Vomiting
   d. Diarrhea
   e. Abdominal discomfort
   f. Headache
   g. Fatigue
   h. Ventricular ectopic beats or bradycardia (irregular or slow pulse)

        i. Blurred vision
        j. A yellow cast to vision or a white halo seen around lights
    10. For a patient receiving digitalis, stress the importance of regular
        serum digitalis measurement, teach the patient how to recognize signs
        and symptoms of digitalis toxicity, and advise the patient to consult the
        physician before taking nonprescription drugs
  D. Evaluation
    1. The patient's arrhythmias are managed successfully through drug
       therapy and treatment of underlying health problems
    2. The patient avoids complications of arrhythmias

IV. Cataracts

  A. General information
    1. A cataract is an opacity in the lens of the eye; usually, cataracts
       develop in both eyes
    2. Cataracts are one of the most common pathologic problems affecting
       the aging eye
    3. The rate of cataract development varies among individuals
    4. Causes of cataracts include:
        a. Normal age-related changes
        b. Traumatic injury to the lens
        c. Changes secondary to other eye disorders or such systemic
           disorders as diabetes, hypoparathyroidism, and atrophic dermatitis
        d. Drug or chemical toxicity from ergot, dinitrophenol, naphthalene,
           or phenothiazines; toxicity from galactose in a patient with
           galactosemia
        e. Congenital defects
    5. The ability to adapt to changes in gradual vision loss varies among
       individuals; factors affecting adaptation include:
        a. Status of the remaining senses
        b. Physical environment
        c. Life-style
        d. Personality
    6. Cataracts potentiate or increase the risk of sensory deprivation in older
       adults
    7. Treatment typically involves surgical cataract extraction (usually done
       on an outpatient basis), with postoperative correction of residual visual
       deficits; surgical procedures include:
        a. Extracapsular cataract extraction (with possible lens implant)
        b. Intracapsular cataract extraction (with possible lens implant)
        c. PHACOEMULSIFICATION

  B. Assessment findings
    1. Signs and symptoms of cataracts vary with cataract location, size and
       degree of the opacity, and presence of other eye abnormalities

2. "Second sight," a phenomenon in which vision improves, may occur in early stages of cataract formation from lens swelling; presbyopic or hyperopic vision may improve and frequent corrective lens prescription changes may be necessary
3. Glare is a predominant complaint in the patient with scattered cataracts, necessitating habitual wearing of tinted or dark glasses to shield the eyes
4. If the cataract is in the center of the lens, vision may improve in dim light when the pupil is dilated widely
5. If the cataract is in the lens periphery, it may not interfere with vision until it grows over the pupil
6. Common complaints in patients with cataracts include:
   a. Poor vision
   b. Eye fatigue
   c. Headache
   d. Increased light sensitivity
   e. Blurred or multiple vision
   f. Difficulty coping with sudden darkness, bright lights, and glare
7. Ophthalmoscopy or slit-lamp examination confirms lens opacity

C. Nursing implications
1. Keep in mind that the nursing goal is to assist the patient to maximize vision
2. Encourage the patient to have regular and frequent eye examinations
3. Expect to administer MYDRIATIC drops to improve vision temporarily
4. Teach the patient the following:
   a. Proper techniques for administering eye drops
   b. Importance of not letting the dropper touch the cornea
   c. Importance of keeping eye drops free from contamination
5. Advise the patient to wear tinted lenses to help cope with glare
6. Assist the patient in planning environmental changes to reduce glare
7. If cataract surgery is scheduled, inform the patient about the nature of surgery, temporary restrictions necessitated by surgery, and the anticipated visual outcome to help the patient plan appropriately
8. As appropriate, teach the patient about postoperative care measures, including:
   a. Protecting the eye by wearing an eye shield
   b. Avoiding activities that increase intraocular pressure (IOP)—for instance, straining at stool, stooping, and lifting heavy objects—because increased IOP puts strain on the suture line
   c. Avoiding rubbing the eye or lying on the operative side
9. Assess for postoperative complications:
   a. Prolapse of the iris (which appears as a bulging wound with a pear-shaped pupil)
   b. HYPHEMA (which manifests as sharp pain in the eye)

   c. Pupillary block glaucoma (which manifests as pain and increased IOP)
   d. UVEITIS (which manifests as pain, photophobia, tearing, and blurred vision)
   10. Assist the patient who did not have a lens implant to adapt to cataract glasses, if prescribed

D. Evaluation
   1. The patient attains maximal vision
   2. The patient demonstrates the proper way to administer eye drops

V. Cerebrovascular accident

A. General information
   1. Cerebrovascular accident (CVA, also called stroke) is characterized by occlusion or hemorrhage of one or more blood vessels in the brain
   2. CVA causes serious damage or ischemia in brain tissues normally perfused by damaged vessels
   3. The risk of CVA increases with age
   4. Conditions that predispose older adults to CVA include hypertension, atherosclerosis, mitral STENOSIS, cardiac disorders, impaired glucose tolerance, anemia, and high serum triglyceride levels
   5. Major types of CVA include thrombotic (blood clot within a blood vessel in the brain or neck), embolic (cerebral embolism), and hemorrhagic (rupture of cerebral blood vessel)
   6. CVA may be classified according to severity
      a. *Transient ischemic attack* (TIA) involves loss of neurologic function caused by abrupt onset of ischemia
         (1) TIA lasts less than 24 hours
         (2) No residual signs occur
      b. *Reversible ischemic neurologic disability* resembles TIA except that the associated neurologic deficit lasts longer (up to 2 days)
      c. A *stroke in evolution* starts as a relatively small neurologic deficit and increases over several hours or days
      d. A *completed stroke* causes neurologic deficits that remain stable for a prolonged period and do not regress completely
   7. Clinical features of CVA vary with the vessel affected, severity of vessel damage, and extent of collateral circulation
   8. If CVA occurs in the left hemisphere of the brain, signs and symptoms affect the right side of the body; if it occurs in the right hemisphere, signs and symptoms affect the left side of the body
   9. CVA resulting in cranial nerve damage causes signs and symptoms of cranial nerve dysfunction on the same side as the CVA
   10. Signs and symptoms of CVA may be obvious or subtle
   11. Recovery from CVA occurs in three stages
       a. Stage 1 is characterized by cerebral edema, which resolves within 4 weeks

      b. Stage 2 is characterized by return of circulation to ischemic areas; some neurologic improvement may occur within 12 weeks

      c. Stage 3 is characterized by possible compensation for lost function by healthy neurons, leading to improvement within 6 months

  12. A patient with right-sided HEMIPLEGIA may be able to function independently with rehabilitation

  13. A patient with left-sided hemiplegia may not be able to maintain an independent life-style because of spatial and perceptual deficits

B. Assessment findings

  1. Signs and symptoms of CVA vary widely and may be subtle

  2. At onset of CVA, the patient may exhibit loss of consciousness, stertorous respirations or a Cheyne-Stokes rhythm, slow pulse rate, increased blood pressure, and rhythmic inflation of one cheek with respiration (if facial paralysis occurs)

      a. The hands and eyes turn toward the injured side of the brain

      b. The swallowing reflex is absent

      c. Deep reflexes in paralyzed limbs are absent

  3. Signs and symptoms of CVA may include hemiplegia, quadriplegia, HEMIANOPIA, urinary and fecal incontinence, sensory loss or alteration, DYSPHASIA, and DYSPHAGIA

  4. With TIA, signs and symptoms may include PARESIS or paralysis of the face or extremities; APHASIA; hemianopia or vision loss in one eye; areas of anesthesia; behavioral or mental changes, including confusion and memory loss; loss of postural tone; vertigo; vomiting; DYSARTHRIA; perioral numbness; visual blurring; and DIPLOPIA

  5. CVA may affect the seven functions described below; severity of the resulting deficits depends on whether the left or right brain hemisphere is damaged

      a. *Language* usually is intact with left-sided hemiplegia; with right-sided hemiplegia, the patient may have varying degrees of receptive and expressive aphasia

      b. *Speech* typically is impaired

         (1) Dysarthria may occur from impaired coordination of speech muscles (usually caused by nerve damage)

         (2) The patient with left-sided hemiplegia may have trouble speaking clearly but does not have difficulty choosing words or understanding speech

         (3) The patient with right-sided hemiplegia may have difficulty speaking and finding the correct words

      c. *Sensory function* may be altered

         (1) With both right- and left-sided hemiplegia, awareness of painful stimuli and temperature may decrease

         (2) Deep pain sensation usually remains intact

         (3) PROPRIOCEPTION may diminish

      (4) HOMONYMOUS HEMIANOPIA may occur on the same side as hemiplegia, or the patient may be unable to see out of either eye in the direction of the paralyzed side

d. *Perception* may be altered
    (1) With left-sided hemiplegia, the patient may lack awareness of the left side of the body and the environment to the left, with or without a visual field deficit
      (a) The patient may ignore stimuli from the left side of the body (unilateral neglect)
      (b) The patient also may have trouble judging depth and vertical and horizontal orientation in the environment
    (2) With right-sided hemiplegia, the patient usually has normal awareness of body and spatial orientation

e. *Movement* typically is impaired
    (1) One side of the body may be paralyzed
    (2) Immediately after CVA, the affected side may become flaccid or limp
    (3) If paralysis persists, the affected side gradually becomes spastic or stiff; facial asymmetry may result
    (4) Speech muscles may be impaired, causing unclear speech and dysphasia
    (5) APRAXIA may occur
      (a) With left-sided hemiplegia, apraxia usually develops on the affected side
      (b) With right-sided hemiplegia, apraxia may be less marked but typically is bilateral

f. *Behavioral style* usually takes on characteristic changes
    (1) Prestroke personality is an important factor in a patient's reaction to CVA
    (2) The patient with left-sided hemiplegia usually overestimates abilities, reacts quickly and impulsively, has a limited attention span and poor concentration, and shows concern over disabilities and the future
    (3) The patient with right-sided hemiplegia usually does not have impaired judgment but commonly underestimates abilities
    (4) Both left- and right-sided hemiplegia cause increased emotional lability, characterized by inappropriate laughter or crying

g. *Memory* deficits are typical after CVA
    (1) Left-sided hemiplegia may cause difficulty remembering new information about the environment, such as location of the call bell
    (2) Right-sided hemiplegia may cause difficulty remembering new information involving language, such as names

6. After CVA, the patient typically experiences grief in coping with functional losses; grieving may recur throughout recovery and rehabilitation
7. A computed tomography (CT) scan shows evidence of thrombotic, embolic, or hemorrhagic CVA or cerebral edema
8. A brain scan indicates ischemic areas (however, the scan may be negative for up to 2 weeks after CVA)
9. Other diagnostic tests may be done to support the diagnosis of CVA
   a. With hemorrhagic CVA, lumbar puncture may reveal blood in cerebrospinal fluid (CSF)
   b. Ophthalmoscopy may reveal signs of hypertension and atherosclerotic changes in retinal arteries
   c. Angiography may indicate the site of blood vessel occlusion or rupture
   d. Electroencephalography may help localize the damaged area

C. Nursing implications
   1. Keep in mind that nursing goals are to prevent deterioration of the patient's condition, to maximize functional abilities, and to help the patient accept physical deficits
   2. Be prepared to carry out appropriate interventions during the acute phase of CVA
      a. Maintain a patent airway and oxygenation
         (1) Position the patient on the side to prevent aspiration
         (2) Suction the airway, as needed and ordered
         (3) Assist with artificial airway insertion and initiation of mechanical ventilation, if appropriate and ordered
      b. Monitor vital signs and neurologic status; report any significant changes to the physician
      c. Maintain fluid and electrolyte balance; administer I.V. fluids, as ordered
   3. Check the patient's gag reflex before providing food or fluids
   4. Administer stool softeners, as ordered, to prevent straining during bowel movements (which increases cerebral pressure)
   5. Provide thorough mouth care
   6. Provide eye care with a cotton ball and sterile normal saline solution; instill eye drops, as ordered and needed
   7. Determine if the patient has language problems, speech problems, or both
   8. Incorporate simple measures into nursing care to allow the patient to communicate basic needs; for instance, use a board containing simple printed requests to which the patient can point
   9. Take measures to prevent or alleviate pain from increased spasticity of the affected side
      a. Perform regular passive range-of-motion exercises
      b. Use proper positioning

      c. Use transfer methods that avoiding putting tension on paralyzed joints
10. Closely supervise the patient with left-sided hemiplegia for unilateral neglect and distortions of depth and vertical/horizontal orientation to prevent injury and to assist with activities of daily living; consistently reinforce awareness of the left side of the body and the physical environment to the patient's left side
11. Prevent injury to paralyzed limbs through proper body positioning and exercises that promote symmetrical posture and movement; consult physical and occupational therapists, as appropriate
12. Provide eating assistance for the dysphagic patient who cannot hold the head up
      a. Elevate the head of the bed at least 45 degrees and turn the patient's head to the unaffected side to promote swallowing
      b. Be aware that semisolid foods are easier to swallow than liquids
13. Prevent injury to the patient with left-sided hemiplegia; caution family and friends that the patient may overestimate abilities
14. Provide encouragement for the patient with right-sided hemiplegia, who is likely to underestimate abilities
15. Assess the patient's functional ability on an ongoing basis to establish realistic, progressive rehabilitation goals
16. Support the patient throughout the grieving process
17. Provide support and teaching about grieving and rehabilitation to members of the patient's support system
18. If speech therapy is indicated, encourage the patient to participate; reinforce such therapy
19. Involve family and friends in the patient's rehabilitation

D. Evaluation
1. The patient attains a maximal level of functioning through rehabilitation therapy
2. The patient adapts to physical deficits successfully while achieving and maintaining maximal life-style independence

VI. Chronic obstructive pulmonary disease

A. General information
1. Chronic obstructive pulmonary disease (COPD) refers to a group of conditions characterized by chronic airway obstruction
2. COPD disorders include chronic bronchitis, chronic emphysema, and asthma, or a combination of these disorders
3. Most older adults with COPD exhibit components of both chronic bronchitis and chronic emphysema
4. COPD is the major cause of respiratory disability in older adults
5. Older adults with COPD are vulnerable to bronchopulmonary infections, which in turn may cause COPD exacerbation

6. Risk factors for COPD include smoking, recurrent or chronic respiratory infections, allergies, and heredity
7. COPD is a progressive disease; the rate of progression varies among individuals

B. Assessment findings
1. Depending on the severity of the disorder, the patient may complain of breathlessness on exertion or dyspnea or shortness of breath at rest
2. Fatigue may occur from the increased work necessary to breathe
3. The patient may cough repeatedly
4. The patient may have trouble sleeping
5. A productive cough may occur intermittently; dyspnea and fatigue on exertion may worsen gradually
6. Anteroposterior chest diameter increases
7. Distant breath sounds may occur from alveolar hyperinflation
8. Wheezing may result from small airway collapse
9. With bronchitis, scattered rhonchi may occur from mucus in the airways
10. Other signs and symptoms of COPD include:
    a. Use of accessory respiratory muscles, especially during expiration
    b. Prolonged expiration
    c. Restlessness or twitching
    d. HYPEREMIA of the hands
    e. Finger clubbing or cyanosis
11. Pulmonary function studies typically show a reduction in the ratio of forced expiratory volume to forced vital capacity measured at 1 second
12. Compensations to COPD commonly develop slowly and insidiously in older adults; for example, arterial blood gas (ABG) values may show a low PaO_2 value and an elevated $PaCO_2$ value, with a pH value near normal from compensatory increases in serum bicarbonate
13. Acutely reduced gas exchange may cause abrupt changes in ABG values and CNS depression

C. Nursing implications
1. Keep in mind that nursing goals are to relieve signs and symptoms of COPD, to prevent complications, and to help the patient adjust to life-style changes
2. Advise the patient to stop smoking and to avoid other respiratory irritants
3. Teach the patient and family about all aspects of the treatment plan; include rationales and instructions for each prescribed medication and therapeutic measure to prepare the patient to assume responsibility for self-care

4. Teach the patient's spouse or caregiver about signs and symptoms indicating onset of disease exacerbation, infection, or respiratory failure (for instance, changes in mentation and judgment, which commonly signal worsening of the patient's condition and warrant medical care)
5. Expect to administer bronchodilators, antibiotics, and steroids
6. Be aware of and teach the patient about side effects of prescribed medications
7. Encourage the patient who does not have heart disease to drink 2 to 3 liters of fluid daily to mobilize secretions; advise the patient to use a humidifier, vaporizer, or nebulizer, if appropriate
8. Perform postural drainage, chest percussion, and vibration to mobilize secretions and improve alveolar ventilation, as ordered; be aware that positions used in maneuvers to drain lung segments can cause harm in older adults
9. Teach the patient proper breathing techniques (such as pursed-lip breathing) to control the rate and depth of respirations
10. Teach the patient how to cough effectively
11. Expect to administer oxygen
12. If oxygen therapy will continue at home, teach the patient and family the purpose of oxygen therapy, proper use and cleaning of oxygen equipment, and signs and symptoms of CO_2 narcosis
13. Encourage the patient to participate in a progressive exercise program, which usually is discussed with the physician and must be carefully planned and supervised
14. Assist the patient in planning and managing life-style changes as COPD progresses
15. Encourage the patient to express feelings and work through grief while adapting to chronic illness
16. Support and assist the patient and family to accept life-style changes

D. Evaluation
   1. The patient adapts to illness as COPD progresses
   2. The patient adapts to life-style changes necessitated by COPD

VII. Congestive heart failure

A. General information
   1. Congestive heart failure (CHF) is a syndrome in which the heart fails to pump effectively; it results in circulatory congestion, pulmonary congestion, or both
   2. Pump failure in the right ventricle is termed *right-sided heart failure;* pump failure in the left ventricle is termed *left-sided heart failure*
   3. Chronic CHF may have an insidious onset because compensatory mechanisms develop in an attempt to maintain adequate cardiac output and perfusion
   4. CHF incidence and prevalence increase with age

5. Older adults with CHF usually have at least one other cardiac disease and other noncardiac health problems
6. Common cardiac diseases associated with CHF in older adults include:
   a. Coronary artery disease
   b. MI
   c. Hypertension associated with cardiac hypertrophy and heart wall stiffness
7. Diseases and disorders that increase the risk of CHF include:
   a. COPD
   b. Pulmonary emboli
   c. Renal disease
   d. Liver disease
   e. Hyperthyroidism
   f. Anemia
8. Other risk factors for CHF include obesity, malnutrition, and a high-sodium diet
9. Drugs that affect cardiac pumping ability or cause sodium and water retention may trigger CHF in older adults
10. Emotional stress and too much or too little physical activity are associated with CHF in older adults
11. Many older adults with CHF can be managed at home with medications, special diet, and modification of exercise and activities of daily living
12. Special considerations in older adults with CHF include their smaller cardiac reserve and increased risk of such disorders as thrombophlebitis, pulmonary emboli, decubitus ulcers, and pneumonia associated with immobility

B. Assessment findings
   1. In older adults, classic signs and symptoms of CHF may be obscured by other diseases
   2. Signs and symptoms of left-sided heart failure include:
      a. Breathlessness
      b. Dyspnea (on exertion or at rest)
      c. Productive cough
      d. Pulmonary congestion
      e. Wheezing
      f. Nocturia
      g. Crackles at the lung bases that do not clear with coughing
   3. Signs and symptoms of right-sided heart failure include:
      a. Edema of the lower extremities
      b. Engorgement of neck veins
      c. Hepatic enlargement and tenderness
      d. Abdominal distention
      e. Anorexia
      f. Nausea

    g. Vomiting

    h. Ascites

    i. Renal insufficiency or oliguria

4. Older adults may exhibit signs and symptoms of both left- and right-sided heart failure

5. Chest pain or tightness may accompany CHF in older adults

6. Diagnostic tests to confirm CHF include:

    a. Chest X-ray taken after full inspiration, which may detect changes in pulmonary vessels and cardiac dilation

    b. Laboratory tests (hepatic enzyme levels, thyroid function, serum electrolyte levels), which may identify precipitating causes of CHF

C. Nursing implications

1. Keep in mind that nursing goals are to decrease the cardiac workload, to increase cardiac output, and to reduce vascular congestion

2. Monitor the patient for signs and symptoms of progressive CHF, such as increasing dyspnea, coughing, or edema

3. Remember that chair rest is preferable to bed rest (if tolerated by the patient)

4. Observe the patient doing simple activities (such as repositioning in bed, eating, washing, and talking) to evaluate activity tolerance

5. Teach the patient to avoid the VALSALVA MANEUVER when repositioning

6. Assist the patient to apply elastic antiembolism stockings, if ordered, to prevent deep-vein thrombosis and emboli

7. Expect to administer diuretics

8. In a patient who is receiving a diuretic, monitor for signs and symptoms of hypokalemia or dehydration, such as weakness, dizziness, and confusion (which may represent diuretic side effects)

9. Weigh the patient daily at the same time and in the same clothing to ensure accurate monitoring of diuresis and edema

10. Expect to administer a cardiac glycoside, such as digitoxin or digoxin

11. In a patient who is receiving digitalis, assess for signs and symptoms of digitalis toxicity, such as anorexia, nausea, vomiting, headache, premature ventricular contractions, and bradycardia; be especially alert for these changes if the patient is receiving both a diuretic and digitalis

12. Teach the patient about the medication regimen and the importance of regularly scheduled laboratory tests (such as serum digitalis, electrolyte, and BUN levels)

13. Advise the patient and family to notify the physician if they notice signs or symptoms of CHF exacerbation, including:

    a. Shortness of breath

    b. Coughing

    c. Edema of the feet, legs, and ankles

    d. Weight gain

14. Expect to administer oxygen therapy

15. If oxygen therapy will continue at home, inform the patient and family of the purpose of such therapy and teach them how to use and clean the equipment

16. Assist the patient in planning daily activities that incorporate rest periods

17. Monitor the patient's emotional responses to the care provided

18. Assist the patient in restricting dietary sodium intake

19. Confirm that the patient understands and follows the sodium-restricted diet

20. Provide emotional support through reassurance and teaching

21. Counsel family members about the patient's need for emotional support and urge them to avoid emotionally stressful interactions with the patient

D. Evaluation
1. The patient's signs and symptoms are managed successfully
2. The patient experiences fewer CHF exacerbations
3. The patient successfully adapts to life-style changes related to diet, medication, and activity level

VIII. Decubitus ulcers

A. General information
1. Decubitus ulcers (pressure sores) result from obstruction of capillary flow that leads to acute tissue ischemia, tissue necrosis, and subsequent ulceration
2. Unrelieved pressure, immobility, and shear forces (friction) contribute to decubitus ulcer formation
3. Factors that place older adults at risk for developing decubitus ulcers include:
    a. Immobility
    b. Impaired sensitivity to pain
    c. Paralysis
    d. Malnutrition
    e. Impaired circulation
    f. Incontinence
    g. Obesity
    h. Edema
    i. Anemia
    j. Confusion
    k. Warm, moist skin areas
4. Immobility is the single greatest risk factor for decubitus ulcer formation
5. Common sites of decubitus ulcer formation include:
    a. Heel
    b. Greater trochanter
    c. Sacrum

      d. Elbow
      e. Scapular spine
      f. Dorsal spine (in thin, kyphotic persons)
  6. Slow healing (from circulatory inadequacy) and increased risk of infection make decubitus ulcers a serious problem for older adults
  7. Nursing intervention at any stage of decubitus ulcer development halts ulcer progression
  8. Enzyme products commonly are used to debride ulcers containing profuse necrotic tissue and eschar
  9. Antibiotic agents reduce the number of bacteria or fungi in a decubitus ulcer

B. Assessment findings
  1. Signs and symptoms of decubitus ulcer vary with the stage of ulcer formation
      a. Stage 1: shiny, erythematous skin over the compressed area
      b. Stage 2: small blisters or erosions
      c. Stage 3: skin breaks, which create a deep pressure sore with tissue involvement
      d. Stage 4: deep pressure sore with tissue, bone, and muscle involvement
  2. Bacteria in the affected area cause inflammation and further necrosis
  3. Black ESCHAR may appear
  4. Foul-smelling, purulent discharge may occur in advanced stages of decubitus ulcer development
  5. Culture and sensitivity testing of exudate from the ulcer identifies organisms present and determines appropriate antibiotics

C. Nursing implications
  1. Keep in mind that the nursing goal is to assist with measures to heal the decubitus ulcer, limit its effects, and prevent recurrence
  2. Identify the high-risk patient and initiate vigorous measures to prevent decubitus ulcer formation
  3. Reposition the immobilized patient at least every 2 hours, depending on the patient's condition
  4. Use alternating air mattresses and padding to prevent or alleviate pressure
  5. Keep the bed clean, dry, and free of wrinkles to help prevent ulcer formation
  6. Provide meticulous skin care, especially if the patient is incontinent; moist skin and feces predispose the perianal area to tissue breakdown and infection
  7. Massage the patient's back and all bony prominences (coccyx, hips, elbows, heels, shoulder blades, knees, and ankles) several times daily, especially when repositioning, to promote circulation

8. Promote healing of decubitus ulcers by providing good nutrition, relieving pressure on the ulcer and bony prominences, promoting good circulation, providing meticulous skin care, and ensuring proper positioning
9. Know that various modalities are used to treat decubitus ulcers, including heat lamp treatments, chemical debridement agents, wet-to-dry dressings, and irrigations and soaks
10. Assist the patient with whirlpool treatments, as ordered, to promote circulation
11. Encourage adequate food and fluid intake to promote optimal healing

D. Evaluation
1. The patient's decubitus ulcer heals successfully
2. The patient avoids further decubitus ulcer formation

IX. Dementia

A. General information
1. Dementia involves permanent, progressive deterioration of mental function and is characterized by confusion, impaired judgment, forgetfulness, and personality changes
2. The most common forms of dementia are multi-infarct dementia and Alzheimer's disease
3. Multi-infarct dementia results from repeated CVAs that cause complete deterioration of cerebral tissue within a circumscribed area
   a. Onset of multi-infarct dementia may be gradual or sudden
   b. Its course is marked by cyclical worsening and improvement of signs and symptoms
   c. The early phase of multi-infarct dementia is characterized by gradual progression of impaired intellectual functioning and partial memory lapses
   d. Delirium may result from insufficient cerebral circulation
4. Alzheimer's disease is characterized by brain atrophy with neurofibrillary tangles, granulovascular changes, neuritic (senile) plaques, and reduced cholinergic enervation
   a. Changes occur gradually, starting with impaired memory and progressing to language and motor changes
   b. The cause of Alzheimer's disease is unknown (see *Possible causes of Alzheimer's disease*, page 72)
   c. Alzheimer's disease progresses in three stages
      (1) Stage 1 lasts from 2 to 4 years
      (2) Stage 2 lasts up to 7 years and is marked by more profound changes and loss of independence
      (3) Stage 3 is terminal and usually does not last longer than 1 year
   d. Duration of Alzheimer's disease is estimated at 5 to 14 years

---

POSSIBLE CAUSES OF ALZHEIMER'S DISEASE

Scientists have proposed various defects as the cause of Alzheimer's disease. The chart below presents several possible causes and rationales.

CAUSE	RATIONALE
Acetylcholine	Direct reduced acetylcholine-mediated transmission of nerve impulses
Genetic	Faulty gene or genes, causing vulnerability to an environmental factor
Toxin	Accumulation of aluminum salts
Abnormal protein	Abnormal protein structures caused by disruption in protein metabolism
Infectious agent	Slow-growing virus of a particular genetic makeup, a concurrent immune disorder, or exposure to an environmental toxin

---

  e. Factors commonly contributing to death in patients with Alzheimer's disease include pneumonia and other infections, malnutrition, and dehydration

B. Assessment findings
 1. The patient with dementia may deny memory loss or make vague complaints of fatigue, dizziness, or occasional headache
 2. The patient may appear in good health except for memory and behavioral changes
 3. The patient may seem fearful and suspicious, clinging to significant others or claiming that misplaced items have been stolen
 4. Signs and symptoms may vary and may progress at different rates from one patient to the next
 5. With multi-infarct dementia, signs and symptoms vary with the brain area affected; they include dizziness, headache, decreased physical and mental vigor, and vague physical complaints
 6. Signs and symptoms of Alzheimer's disease vary with the disease stage
  a. During stage 1, signs and symptoms include spatial and time disorientation, inappropriate affect, and decreased concentration
   (1) The patient exhibits transient paranoia, careless dressing or grooming, impaired judgment, and perceptual disturbances
   (2) Forgetfulness and memory loss occur
  b. During stage 2, signs and symptoms include inability to recognize familiar persons or to interpret the environment, ASTEREOGNOSIS, poor comprehension, and complete disorientation
   (1) HYPERTONIA, nocturnal restlessness, apraxia, wandering, and hoarding are other prominent features

---

DRUGS USED FOR PATIENTS WITH ALZHEIMER'S DISEASE

Prescription drugs are used to treat behavioral manifestations of the disease. No drug has been shown to reverse the pathology of the disease. The chart below lists some of the drugs used for control of cognitive and affective symptoms. Drugs currently under investigation include pentylenetetrazole and tacrine.

SYMPTOMS	DRUG	COMMENTS
Cognitive symptoms	• Ergotoid mesylates (dihydroergotoxine)	• Approved 15 to 29 years ago (combination of ergo & alkaloids) • May have mild mood-elevating effect.
	• Papaverine • Isoxsurpine • Cyclandelate	• Used for their vasodilating effect
	• Methylphenidate • Pentylenetetrazole	• Used for their stimulant effect
	• Tacrine	• Used to treat memory loss and dementia
	• Thioridazine • Haloperidol	• Used to treat psychotic symptoms • Haloperidol not recommended for aging adults because of possible adverse reactions of sedation and increasing confusion.
Affective symptoms	• Nortriptyline • Desipramine	• Used for antidepressant action
	• Trazodone HCl • Diphenhydramine	• Used for sedative effect • Hypnotic action; used to treat sleep deficits

    (2) The patient has a ravenous appetite without weight gain, is unable to read or write, has problems communicating, and exhibits short- and long-term memory loss

  c. During stage 3, the patient becomes totally dependent

    (1) PARAPHASIA, irritability, blank facial expression, hyperorality, seizures, appetite loss, and emaciation are common

    (2) The patient is unable to recognize family members

7. Laboratory tests, such as complete blood count, VDRL (Venereal Disease Research Laboratory) test, serum electrolyte levels, and thyroid studies, are ordered to rule out treatable causes of dementia

8. A thorough drug history is obtained to rule out drug-induced dementia

9. A mental status examination is performed to rule out depression (see *Folstein mini-mental state examination*, page 74)

FOLSTEIN MINI-MENTAL STATE EXAMINATION

The Folstein Mini-Mental State Examination is the preferred tool for assessing the mental status of a patient with suspected cognitive impairment. To perform the examination, ask the patient to follow a series of simple commands that test his ability to understand and perform cognitive functions. Award a designated point value for successful completion of each instruction; then total the scores to determine the patient's mental status. Scores of 26 to 30 indicate that the patient is normal; 22 to 25, mildly impaired; and less than 22; significantly impaired.

PATIENT INSTRUCTIONS	MAXIMUM SCORE	ACTUAL SCORE
Orientation		
• Ask the patient to name the year, season, date, day, and month. (Score one point for each correct response.)	5	( )
• Ask the patient to name his state, city, street, and house address, and the room in which he is standing. (Score one point for each correct response.)	5	( )
Comprehension		
Name three objects, pausing 1 second between each name. Then ask the patient to repeat all three names. (Score one point for each correct response.) Repeat this exercise until the patient can correctly name all three objects (the patient will be tested on his ability to recall this information later in the examination).	3	( )
Attention and calculation		
Ask the patient to count backward by sevens, beginning at 100; have him stop after counting out five numbers. Alternatively, ask the patient to spell "World" backward. (Score one point for each correct response.)	5	( )
Recall		
Ask the patient to restate the name of the three objects previously identified in the examination. (Score one point for each correct response.)	3	( )
Language		
• Point to a pencil and a watch. Ask the patient to identify each object. (Score one point for each correct response.)	2	( )
• Ask the patient to repeat "No ifs, ands, or buts." (Score one point for a correct response.)	1	( )
• Ask the patient to take a paper in his right hand, then fold the paper in half, then put the paper on the floor. (Score one point for each correct response to this three-part command.)	3	( )

(continued)

FOLSTEIN MINI-MENTAL STATE EXAMINATION *(continued)*

PATIENT INSTRUCTIONS	MAXIMUM SCORE	ACTUAL SCORE
Language *(continued)*		
● Ask the patient to read and obey the written instruction "Close your eyes." (Score one point for a correct response.)	1	( )
● Ask the patient to copy the following design. (Score one point for a correct response.)	1	( )

Adapted with permission from Folstein, M.F., et al. "Mini-Mental State: A Practical Method for Grading the Cognitive State of Patients for the Clinician," *Journal of Psychiatric Research* 12:196-97, 1975.

---

10. Thorough physical, neurologic, and psychiatric examinations are conducted to rule out other disorders with similar clinical features
11. A CT scan may show evidence of CVA, multi-infarct dementia, tumor, changes in CSF flow, hematoma, or cerebral atrophy
12. Positron emission tomography, which measures metabolic activity of the cerebral cortex, may be used to distinguish Alzheimer's disease from other forms of dementia
13. Postmortem brain biopsy is the only definitive diagnostic test for Alzheimer's disease; otherwise, provisional diagnosis is made after excluding other causes of dementia

C. Nursing implications
1. Keep in mind that nursing goals are to help the patient maintain optimal health, to protect the patient from injury, and to provide physical and intellectual stimulation
2. Assist the patient who has memory deficits by incorporating reality orientation as an ongoing process during all nursing interventions
3. Reassure the patient who overreacts to unfamiliar situations by speaking calmly and slowly and by reducing environmental distractions
4. Offer support and recognize the patient's feelings as the patient tries to cope with loss of personal finances and independence, employment difficulties, and inability to drive a car or perform simple daily activities

5. Offer support to family members and caregivers by describing disease progression, teaching them how to alleviate the patient's signs and symptoms, and referring them to community resources and support groups
6. Assist the family and caregivers in managing problems related to the patient's wandering, eating, toileting, and inappropriate behavior
7. Protect the patient from injury by teaching the family and caregivers to identify and correct potential safety hazards

D. Evaluation
1. The patient's behavioral and personality changes are managed successfully
2. The patient, family members, and caregivers demonstrate an understanding of coping strategies and community resources

X. Diabetes mellitus

A. General information
1. Diabetes mellitus is a chronic disease of carbohydrate metabolism in which insulin is deficient or target tissue is resistant to insulin (insulin resistance renders insulin ineffective)
2. The disease is characterized by hyperglycemia, insulin deficiency or resistance, and premature degenerative changes in the CNS and circulatory system
3. Types of diabetes mellitus include insulin-dependent and non-insulin-dependent diabetes mellitus
   a. Insulin-dependent diabetes mellitus (IDDM, or Type I)
      (1) This disease usually occurs before age 25 but may develop in older adults
      (2) It is characterized by little or no insulin production
   b. Non-insulin-dependent diabetes mellitus (NIDDM, or Type II)
      (1) This disease usually develops after age 40
      (2) It is common in older adults
      (3) Insulin is produced but may be insufficient or ineffective in preventing hyperglycemia
4. Glucose intolerance (impaired ability to metabolize glucose) in older adults may result from age-related changes in insulin levels and insulin release, decreased peripheral effectiveness of insulin, or a combination of these factors
5. Acute illness increases insulin demand
6. Decreased exercise levels in older adults may contribute to glucose intolerance
7. Medications commonly taken by older adults (such as thiazide diuretics, furosemide, ethacrynic acid, nicotinic acid, estrogen, cortisone, and levodopa) also may contribute to glucose intolerance
8. Atherosclerotic cardiovascular disease may develop prematurely in patients with diabetes mellitus

9. Risk factors for diabetes mellitus include heredity, obesity, and prolonged elevation of stress hormone levels (cortisol, epinephrine, glucagon, and growth hormone) from physiologic or emotional stress

10. Older adults with newly diagnosed diabetes mellitus commonly are managed by a low-calorie diabetic diet

11. Older adults with diabetes are predisposed to:
    a. Urinary tract infection
    b. Foot and leg ulcers
    c. Pruritus
    d. Recurrent skin infections
    e. Vaginitis and sexual dysfunction (women)
    f. Chronic impotence (men)

12. Acute complications of diabetes and its treatment are serious problems in older adults, necessitating prompt intervention to prevent further morbidity or death; such complications include diabetic ketoacidosis, hyperglycemic nonketotic hyperosmolar coma, and hypoglycemia

13. Long-term complications of diabetes mellitus include:
    a. Vascular disease
    b. Atherosclerosis
    c. Diabetic retinopathy
    d. Peripheral and autonomic neuropathy
    e. Nephropathy

B. Assessment findings
   1. Older adults with diabetes mellitus may be asymptomatic
   2. Classic signs and symptoms of hyperglycemia, such as POLYURIA, POLYDIPSIA, POLYPHAGIA, and weight loss, may be absent in older adults
   3. Signs and symptoms of hyperglycemia in older adults may include fatigue, infection, and evidence of neuropathy (such as sensory changes)
   4. Sudden weight gain commonly precedes diabetes in older adults
   5. The urine glucose level may not be an accurate indicator of elevated blood glucose in older adults because of their increased threshold for urinary glucose excretion
   6. Laboratory findings that suggest diabetes mellitus include a fasting blood glucose level above 140 mg/dl, confirmed by a second test, and an oral glucose tolerance test using age-corrected norms

C. Nursing implications
   1. Keep in mind that the nursing goal is to assist the patient with life-style changes to control diabetes and limit its effects
   2. Help the patient modify the diet to meet medical requirements and satisfy personal preferences
   3. Expect to administer insulin or oral hypoglycemic medications
   4. Observe for signs and symptoms of a hypoglycemic reaction, such as tremors, diaphoresis, tachycardia, and altered level of consciousness
   5. Teach the patient about the following:

    a. Self-testing of blood or urine glucose
    b. Prescribed dietary changes
    c. Insulin administration, if prescribed
    d. Oral hypoglycemic agents, if prescribed
    e. Hypoglycemic reactions
    f. Care during concurrent illness
    g. Foot care

6. Evaluate the patient's ability to draw up the correct insulin dosage and administer the injection safely
7. Provide the patient with a written medication schedule
8. Assist the patient in planning an individualized exercise program
9. Teach the patient to perform mouth care twice daily to prevent fungal infections that may occur under dentures and at the corners of the mouth (common in diabetic patients)
10. Teach the patient how to perform proper foot care and daily foot inspection; stress the importance of such care
11. Teach the patient to avoid conditions that impair circulation, such as smoking, leg crossing, a cold environment, tight-fitting clothing, knee-length hose, and furniture that presses against the calf or back of the knee
12. Teach the patient the importance of proper daily skin care; stress the need to avoid complications caused by extreme temperatures, irritation, trauma, and infection
13. Advise the patient with newly diagnosed diabetes to have an ophthalmologic examination

D. Evaluation
1. The patient's serum glucose level remains within a normal range (adjusted for age)
2. The patient adapts successfully to the therapeutic regimen
3. The patient's disease complications are managed successfully

XI. Diverticular disease

A. General information
1. Diverticular disease is the most common colon disease in the Western world; it may occur as diverticulosis or diverticulitis
2. Diverticulosis, usually an asymptomatic disorder, is characterized by diverticula, saclike herniations of the mucous membrane that push through intestinal muscle fibers
3. Diverticula usually begin to develop around age 50, increasing in size and number with age
4. Diverticulosis affects an estimated 40% of persons over age 70
5. Risk factors for diverticulosis include:
    a. Aging
    b. Obesity
    c. History of constipation

      d. Hiatal hernia
      e. History of a diet high in refined, low-residue foods
      f. Emotional stress
  6. Diverticulitis (inflammation of diverticula) is a serious complication in older adults with diverticulosis; precipitating factors for diverticulitis include:
      a. Obesity
      b. Consumption of alcohol or irritating foods
      c. Excessive coughing
      d. Straining at stool
  7. Possible complications of diverticulitis include:
      a. Intestinal perforation
      b. Severe intestinal bleeding
      c. Peritonitis
      d. Intestinal abscesses
      e. Intestinal fistulae
      f. Obstruction
  8. Treatment of diverticular disease depends on the severity of symptoms
  9. Older adults can benefit from measures to prevent diverticular disease, such as eating a high-fiber diet and preventing constipation
 10. Careful investigation of GI complaints in older adults is important to rule out more serious disorders, such as colon cancer

B. Assessment findings
  1. Some persons with diverticulosis are asymptomatic
  2. Signs and symptoms of diverticulosis may include:
      a. Change in bowel habits (usually constipation or diarrhea, or constipation alternating with diarrhea)
      b. Tenderness or pain in the lower left quadrant that increases in severity at a consistent interval after meals or after emotional disturbance
  3. Signs and symptoms of diverticulitis may range from mild to severe with sudden onset; they may include:
      a. Abdominal pain
      b. Chills
      c. Fever
      d. Nausea
      e. Rebound tenderness
      f. Rectal bleeding
  4. Results of a barium enema may reveal spasms in muscles around diverticula; spasms cause narrowing, obstruction, hypermotility, and other changes in the colon
  5. Sigmoidoscopy and flexible colonoscopy may reveal colonic irritability and spasm

C. Nursing implications
 1. Keep in mind that nursing goals are to relieve signs and symptoms and to prevent recurrence and complications of diverticular disease
 2. Be aware that for a patient with acute diverticulitis, nursing interventions may include:
    a. Promoting bed rest
    b. Giving fluids only, or withholding food and fluids, as ordered
    c. Administering I.V. therapy to maintain fluid and electrolyte balance, as ordered
    d. Stressing the importance of progressing from a low-residue to a high-residue diet
    e. Administering blood replacement products, as ordered, if bleeding is present
    f. Administering analgesics, sedatives, spasmolytic agents, antibiotics, or local heat, as ordered
 3. Teach the patient the importance of consuming a high-fiber diet to manage and prevent diverticular disease
 4. Be aware that a high-fiber diet may cause special problems in older adults, such as:
    a. Inclusion of more food than the patient reasonably can ingest
    b. Eating problems caused by poor tooth condition or ill-fitting dentures
    c. Flatulence, distention, or diarrhea
 5. Emphasize the importance of preventing or relieving constipation
 6. Teach measures to prevent constipation, such as:
    a. Maintaining a high fluid intake to soften stools
    b. Increasing daily exercise, if possible
 7. Avoid using a bed pan for the patient, if possible; instead, assist the patient to the toilet or bedside commode to promote proper positioning and abdominal muscle use during bowel movements
 8. Provide privacy and an unhurried atmosphere while the patient uses the toilet

D. Evaluation
 1. The patient avoids or experiences relief from signs and symptoms of diverticular disease
 2. The patient expresses a need for daily exercise

XII. Fractures

A. General information
 1. A fracture is a partial or complete disruption in bone continuity
 2. The risk of sustaining a serious fracture increases after age 40
 3. Older adults are more susceptible to fractures from even minimal forces because of a high incidence of osteoporosis, osteomalacia, and age-related bone loss

4. Such age-related changes as weakened muscles, tendons, and cartilage also increase the incidence of fractures in older adults

5. Common chronic conditions in older adults (such as arthritis, cataracts, glaucoma, and neurologic problems affecting gait or limiting vision or mobility) may increase the risk of falls and fractures

6. In older adults, fractures usually occur in cancellous bone near joints (in younger persons, the bone shaft is the typical fracture site)

7. Fractures are more common in older adult women than older adult men

8. The percentage of falls resulting in fractures increases with age

9. The most common fracture sites in older adults are:
   a. Vertebrae
   b. Upper end of the femur (hip fracture)
   c. Distal end of the radius (Colles' fracture)
   d. Proximal end of the humerus

10. The most common and potentially most disabling fractures are those of the upper end of the femur

11. Fractures of the femoral neck carry the greatest risk of nonunion and posttraumatic degenerative joint disease because blood supply to the femoral head runs through the femoral neck

12. Older adult women living alone have the highest risk for hip fracture

13. For older adults, successful recovery from a fracture depends on avoiding complications, such as:
    a. Permanent disability
    b. Joint contractures
    c. Skin breakdown
    d. Fat emboli syndrome
    e. Pulmonary emboli
    f. Nerve damage

14. Fractures should be treated promptly; untreated or inadequately treated fractures may cause permanent disability and dependency

15. Treatment for a hip fracture may involve such surgical procedures as open or closed internal fixation and total hip replacement

B. Assessment findings
   1. Signs and symptoms of a fracture depend on the location, severity, and type of fracture and length of the interval before treatment begins
   2. For all types of fractures, signs and symptoms may include:
      a. Pain
      b. Inability to move the injured part
      c. Pallor
      d. Ecchymosis
      e. Tenderness localized to a specific point
      f. Paresthesia
      g. Edema
      h. Deformity

      i. CREPITUS
      j. Confusion
  3. With hip fracture, specific signs and symptoms vary with the fracture location; however, the affected limb usually shows:
      a. Shortening
      b. Flexion
      c. Weakness
      d. External foot rotation
      e. Pain at the knee, fracture site, or both (however, pain may be absent)
  4. Dehydration, skin breakdown, and hypothermia may occur in the older adult who is alone at the time of injury and is not found for several hours
  5. X-rays of the affected area show the location, extent, and severity of the fracture
  6. For the patient with a hip fracture, the physician may order a complete blood count, blood type and cross-matching, serum electrolyte measurement, and prothrombin and partial thromboplastin times
  7. Neurovascular assessment of the area distal to the fracture helps detect any vascular or nerve damage

C. Nursing implications
  1. Keep in mind that nursing goals are to promote rehabilitation, to limit immobility, to prevent complications, and to prevent the patient from falling again
  2. Assist with fracture immobilization, as appropriate
  3. Perform frequent neurovascular assessments of the area distal to the fracture
  4. Provide meticulous care to all exposed skin around the injury site
  5. Teach the patient about proper cast care, if appropriate
  6. Assist with an exercise program to prevent immobility
  7. Provide patient teaching to prevent falls by:
      a. Helping the patient identify and correct any home safety hazards
      b. Cautioning the patient not to perform activities that increase the risk of a fall (such as vacuuming) when taking medications that cause drowsiness
      c. Encouraging the patient to be alert for environmental hazards that can cause falls, such as wet floors and loose carpets
      d. Warning the patient not to go outside in icy weather, if possible
      e. Helping the patient identify behaviors that increase the risk of falling, such as rushing to answer the telephone
      f. Helping the patient overcome the fear of falling by using the prevention techniques described above

D. Evaluation
  1. The patient successfully recovers from the fracture with no residual disability

2. The patient demonstrates an understanding of how to prevent falls

XIII. Glaucoma

A. General information
1. Glaucoma is a collective term for a group of disorders characterized by increased IOP, which can damage the optic nerve
2. Three forms of glaucoma typically occur in older adults:
   a. Acute (angle-closure) glaucoma, characterized by acute onset of increased IOP from narrowing of the anterior chamber angle
   b. Chronic open-angle glaucoma, characterized by insidious onset of increased IOP from a defect in aqueous humor outflow
   c. Chronic closed-angle glaucoma, characterized by insidious onset of increased IOP from narrowing of the anterior chamber angle
3. Chronic open-angle glaucoma is the most common form of glaucoma in older adults, accounting for about 90% of glaucoma cases; it exhibits a hereditary tendency
4. Lens thickening, a result of aging, can lead to a shallow anterior chamber, predisposing an older adult to glaucoma
5. Untreated glaucoma can lead to vision loss and blindness

B. Assessment findings
1. Signs and symptoms depend on the glaucoma form
2. Chronic open-angle glaucoma usually is bilateral and takes a slowly progressive course; signs and symptoms appear late in the disease and include:
   a. Mild aching in the eyes
   b. Loss of peripheral vision
   c. Halos seen around lights
   d. Reduced visual acuity (especially at night)
   e. Headaches
3. Chronic closed-angle glaucoma can be unilateral or bilateral and is characterized by intermittent episodes of increased IOP that resolve spontaneously; signs and symptoms resemble those of chronic open-angle glaucoma
4. Acute closed-angle glaucoma is unilateral; signs and symptoms include:
   a. Excruciating pain
   b. Nausea and vomiting
   c. Inflammation
   d. Halos seen around lights
   e. Dilated pupil that is nonreactive to light
   f. Globe that feels hard to the touch
   g. Cloudy cornea
5. Diagnostic tests that help confirm glaucoma include tonometry to measure IOP, slit-lamp examination of anterior eye structures, and gonioscopy to measure the anterior chamber angle

C. Nursing implications
   1. Keep in mind that the nursing goal is to prevent vision loss
   2. Encourage older adults to have yearly eye examinations that include IOP measurement
   3. For chronic open-angle glaucoma, expect to administer eye drops to decrease aqueous humor production or MIOTICS (such as pilocarpine) to promote aqueous humor outflow
   4. Be aware that chronic glaucoma can be treated with argon laser trabeculoplasty or trabeculectomy and iridectomy
   5. For acute closed-angle glaucoma, expect to administer timolol maleate (Timoptic Solution), miotic eye drops, I.V. medications (such as a carbonic anhydrase inhibitor or a hyperosmotic agent to decrease IOP rapidly by reducing aqueous humor formation), and pain medication; if drugs fail to reduce IOP, expect the patient to undergo laser surgery or iridectomy
   6. Teach the patient how to administer eye drops and how to recognize side effects of prescribed medications
   7. Stress the importance of meticulous daily compliance with prescribed drug therapy to reduce or prevent increased IOP

D. Evaluation
   1. The patient's IOP decreases
   2. The patient understands the importance of drug therapy

XIV. Hypertension

A. General information
   1. Hypertension refers to a persistent elevation in diastolic or systolic blood pressure above that considered normal for the patient's age
   2. Controversy exists over what constitutes normal blood pressure and hypertension in older adults
   3. Age-related changes that may contribute to hypertension in older adults include:
      a. Aortic rigidity
      b. Decreased baroreceptor sensitivity
      c. Decreased arteriolar lumen size
      d. Reduced GFR
      e. Changes in the renin-angiotensin system
      f. Hormonal and cardiovascular changes
   4. Risk factors for hypertension include:
      a. Heredity
      b. Obesity
      c. Stress
      d. Diet high in sodium or saturated fats
      e. Cigarette smoking
      f. Sedentary life-style

5. Hypertension is a major risk factor for cardiovascular disease in older adults, predisposing them to cerebrovascular accident, cardiac disease, and renal failure
6. Systolic blood pressure takes longer to return to resting levels after exercise in older adults than in younger persons
7. Up to age 70, systolic and diastolic blood pressure increase slightly in both men and women
8. In women over age 70, systolic blood pressure may decrease slightly
9. In older adults, systolic pressure may increase more rapidly than diastolic pressure, causing widened PULSE PRESSURE
10. Hypertension occurs in two forms
    a. Essential (idiopathic or primary) hypertension, which has no identifiable cause and may be multifactorial in origin
    b. Secondary hypertension, which results from an underlying cause
11. Isolated systolic hypertension (an increase in systolic pressure without an increase in diastolic pressure) in older adults may result from:
    a. Severe anemia
    b. Paget's disease
    c. Thyrotoxicosis
    d. Aortic regurgitation
12. After age 60, diastolic hypertension may occur when a thrombus or embolus develops in an atherosclerotic lesion in a renal artery
13. Controversy exists over which type of treatment is appropriate in older adults

B. Assessment findings
    1. The patient may be asymptomatic
    2. Signs and symptoms of hypertension include:
        a. Dull headache on awakening
        b. Impaired memory
        c. Nausea and vomiting
        d. Epistaxis
        e. Slow tremor
    3. In many cases, diagnosis in adults over age 50 rests on a blood pressure elevation above 150/95 mm Hg, measured on three separate occasions

C. Nursing implications
    1. Keep in mind that the nursing goal is to reduce the patient's blood pressure gradually to the goal set by the physician
    2. Measure blood pressure with the patient in at least two different positions – lying or sitting and standing – to detect postural blood pressure changes
    3. Help the patient reduce sodium intake through teaching and meal planning; explain how to read food packaging labels to determine the sodium content

4. Promote a restful and nonstressful environment; encourage regular exercise
5. Assist in a weight reduction plan if the patient is obese
6. Teach the patient about prescribed antihypertensive medications; instruct the patient how to prevent and manage a hypotensive reaction by:
    a. Moving slowly from a sitting or lying position
    b. Avoiding standing motionless, taking hot baths, and consuming excessive alcohol
    c. Using caution when driving within 2 hours after taking antihypertensive medication
    d. Lying down with feet elevated to increase cerebral blood flow if hypotension occurs
7. Stress the importance of potassium replacement for a patient who is receiving a thiazide diuretic
8. Be aware that adrenergic blocking agents may cause sudden blood pressure changes because their action is less predictable and harder to control in older adults
9. Assess for side effects of antihypertensive medications that may mimic such age-related problems as dizziness, impaired vision, and difficulty walking

D. Evaluation
1. The patient achieves and maintains goal blood pressure
2. The patient avoids hypertensive crisis

XV. Hypothyroidism

A. General information
1. Hypothyroidism is a state of low serum thyroid hormone and its effect on body tissues
2. The disorder usually occurs after age 50
3. Possible causes of inadequate serum thyroid hormone include:
    a. Thyroid gland dysfunction resulting from surgery, radiation therapy, inflammation, chronic immune thyroiditis (Hashimoto's disease), or such inflammatory conditions as amyloidosis and sarcoidosis
    b. Pituitary failure to produce thyroid-stimulating hormone (TSH)
    c. Hypothalamic failure to produce thyrotropin-releasing hormone (TRH)
    d. Iodine deficiency (usually dietary)
    e. Antithyroid medications prescribed to treat thyrotoxicosis
4. Hypothyroidism may have an insidious onset, preventing or delaying diagnosis in older adults
5. In older adults, hypothyroidism occurs in varying degrees

6. Older adults with hypothyroidism are at greater risk for myxedema coma, a life-threatening and advanced disease stage; myxedema coma usually occurs in patients with preexisting or undiagnosed hypothyroidism after such precipitating factors as infection, trauma, and use of drugs that suppress the CNS
7. Hypothyroidism is treated by thyroid hormone replacement
8. Increased cholesterol levels, atherosclerosis, and coronary disease are common in older adults with hypothyroidism
9. Weakening of the cardiac muscle (a normal age-related change) makes older adults with hypothyroidism susceptible to coronary insufficiency, CHF, and cardiac arrest—especially after overly vigorous thyroid hormone replacement therapy

B. Assessment findings
1. In older adults, clinical features of hypothyroidism resemble—and may be masked by—normal age-related changes, complicating detection of the disorder
2. Signs and symptoms of hypothyroidism include:
   a. Changes in mental status, such as apathy, forgetfulness, and sleepiness, which may be mistaken for ordinary confusion
   b. Metabolic abnormalities, such as cold intolerance, weakness, lassitude, and low energy
   c. Circulatory impairment, manifested by such problems as decreases in cardiac output, heart rate, and blood pressure
   d. Respiratory problems, such as decreased respiratory rate and dyspnea on exertion
   e. GI signs, such as weight gain, constipation, and poor appetite
   f. Sluggish motor activity with hypoactive reflexes
3. Changes in general appearance may include dry thickened skin, sparse dry hair, brittle nails, and anemia
4. The patient may bruise easily and show signs of nonpitting edema (putty face, hands, and feet)
5. Radioimmunoassay reveals low serum levels of triiodothyronine (T_3) and thyroxine (T_4)
6. TSH levels may be increased from thyroid insufficiency or decreased from hypothalamic or pituitary insufficiency
7. Serum cholesterol, alkaline phosphatase, and triglyceride levels may be elevated
8. Normocytic normochromic anemia may be present
9. In myxedema coma, laboratory tests may show a decreased serum sodium level and ABG analysis may reveal decreased pH and increased $PaCO_2$ values, signalling respiratory acidosis from a decreased respiratory rate
10. Signs and symptoms of myxedema coma include:
    a. Hypothermia
    b. Hypoventilation

    c. Hypotension
    d. Hypoactive reflexes
    e. Bradycardia
    f. Cool, dry skin
    g. Seizures
    h. Edema of the face (especially the periorbital region) and extremities
    i. Decreased level of consciousness, ranging from slow mentation to stupor and coma

C. Nursing implications
1. Keep in mind that the nursing goal is to provide support and comfort while taking measures to restore euthyroidism (normal thyroid function)
2. Know that unduly aggressive treatment of hypothyroidism can cause adverse cardiac effects, such as chest pain and tachycardia
3. Assess the patient for signs and symptoms of hyperthyroidism during thyroid hormone replacement therapy
4. Stay alert for hypertension and CHF in the older adult receiving thyroid hormone replacement therapy
5. Caution the patient that abrupt withdrawal of thyroid hormone replacement therapy may precipitate myxedema coma
6. Be aware that an infection may precipitate myxedema coma; check for possible infectious sources, such as in blood, urine, and sputum
7. Know that nursing interventions during myxedema coma include:
    a. Monitoring vital signs, fluid intake and output, ABG results, and serum electrolyte levels
    b. Providing skin care and turning the bedridden patient at least every 2 hours
    c. Maintaining a patent I.V. line
    d. Avoiding sedation, if possible, or reducing the dosage of a prescribed sedative, as ordered
    e. Providing oxygen or mechanical ventilation for respiratory assistance, as appropriate and ordered
    f. Administering I.V. thyroid hormone, if ordered
8. Teach the patient the importance of seeking prompt medical attention for infections
9. Instruct the patient to report chest pain and tachycardia promptly
10. Provide a warm environment and adequate clothing during thyroid hormone replacement therapy
11. Consider the patient's limitations when planning activities
12. Promote good nutrition and prevent constipation by providing a high-protein, low-calorie, high-fiber diet
13. Apply lotion to the patient's skin if it is dry
14. Teach the patient and family the importance of continued treatment and medical supervision

D. Evaluation
   1. The patient regains and maintains a euthyroid state
   2. The patient and family demonstrate an understanding of signs and symptoms of medication overdose, the hazards of therapeutic noncompliance, and the need for lifetime thyroid hormone replacement therapy

XVI. Myocardial infarction

A. General information
   1. Myocardial infarction (MI) refers to occlusion of a coronary artery resulting in severe myocardial ischemia and necrosis
   2. The mortality rate from MI is twice as high in persons over age 70 as in younger persons
   3. Age-related changes in blood, vessel walls, and hemodynamics increase the risk of MI in older adults
   4. Physical exertion or ingestion of a large meal may precipitate MI in susceptible older adults
   5. MI occurs in men and women at approximately equal rates
   6. Risk factors for MI include:
      a. Family history
      b. Hypertension
      c. Obesity
      d. Diabetes mellitus
      e. Smoking
      f. Stress
      g. Sedentary life-style
      h. High serum cholesterol and/or triglyceride levels
   7. Silent MI (MI with no apparent signs or symptoms) is common in older adults and may cause sudden death
   8. Older adults with MI are at risk for such complications as:
      a. Serious arrhythmias
      b. CHF
      c. Cardiogenic shock
      d. Digitalis toxicity (with digitalis therapy)
      e. Cardiac rupture

B. Assessment findings
   1. Signs and symptoms of MI typically are subtle and variable; in older adults, they include:
      a. Dyspnea
      b. Sudden mental deterioration
      c. Dizziness
      d. Intense, prolonged weakness and fatigue
      e. Feeling of faintness
      f. Loss of consciousness
      g. Abdominal distress

        h. Vomiting
        i. Hiccups
        j. Palpitations
    2. In some older adults, pain and other signs and symptoms may be absent
    3. In older adults, MI may cause progressive renal failure with uremia, or embolic occlusion of noncerebral arteries with ischemia or peripheral gangrene
    4. ECG may show an elevated ST segment and inverted T waves; however, ECG changes may be hard to interpret because of possible preexisting cardiac disease
    5. Laboratory test results suggesting MI include elevated serum glutamicoxaloacetic transaminase, lactic dehydrogenase, and creatine phosphokinase levels

C. Nursing implications
    1. Keep in mind that the nursing goal is to decrease the cardiac workload
    2. Assess the patient for pain and administer analgesics, as ordered; monitor for side effects of medications
    3. Expect to administer sedatives; however, be aware that sedatives may cause psychosis and sensory deprivation in older adults (especially those in coronary care units) and may lead to feeding problems, increasing the risk of aspiration pneumonia
    4. Assist with and monitor the patient's exercise; keep in mind that short periods of chair rest are preferable to bed rest
    5. Observe for signs and symptoms of systemic or pulmonary embolism and venous thrombosis
    6. Expect to administer anticoagulants; carefully assess for bleeding
    7. Provide psychosocial support and teaching about MI and rehabilitation to the patient and family
    8. Teach the patient the importance of progressive cardiac rehabilitation
    9. Make sure the patient understands the prescribed activity plan and medications and the importance of follow-up medical care

D. Evaluation
    1. The patient recovers from MI
    2. The patient successfully adapts to life-style changes necessitated by MI

XVII. Osteoarthritis

A. General information
    1. Osteoarthritis is a nonsystemic joint disease that affects mainly older adults
    2. It is characterized by breakdown of articular cartilage with bone hypertrophy at the margins and synovial membrane changes

3. Osteoarthritis is classified as primary (idiopathic) or secondary (caused by other conditions)
4. Sites most commonly affected by osteoarthritis include:
   a. Hip joint
   b. Knee
   c. Distal interphalangeal joints
   d. Proximal interphalangeal joints
   e. Cervical spine
   f. Lumbosacral spine
5. Factors that influence osteoarthritis progression include:
   a. Aging
   b. Trauma
   c. Obesity
   d. Heredity
   e. Prior inflammatory disease
   f. Metabolic and endocrine disorders
6. Osteoarthritis usually progresses slowly
7. Discomfort and stiffness may cause progressive immobilization in older adults and disrupt or restrict daily activities and life-style

B. Assessment findings
   1. Signs and symptoms of osteoarthritis vary from mild to severe, depending on the degree of joint degeneration
   2. Aching joint pain and stiffness usually increase after overuse or inactivity
   3. Pain and stiffness brought on by activity commonly are relieved by rest
   4. Stiffness on awakening or after inactivity usually subsides with exercise or activity
   5. Loss of joint mobility and stiffness may make even simple movements painful
   6. Posture and gait abnormalities may stem from muscle weakness
   7. Crepitus may be heard when roughened articular or extra-articular surfaces contact each other
   8. X-rays typically reveal:
      a. Narrowing of the joint space
      b. Bony changes
      c. Formation of nodes (enlargements) on distal interphalangeal finger joints (Heberden nodes) or proximal interphalangeal finger joints (Bouchard's nodes)

C. Nursing implications
   1. Keep in mind that nursing goals are to relieve discomfort, to maintain range of motion, and to prevent crippling deformities
   2. If the patient is receiving aspirin, stay alert for such side effects as tinnitus, GI upset, and occult blood loss

3. If the patient is receiving nonsteroidal anti-inflammatory agents, teach about potential side effects, such as GI upset
4. Be aware that physical therapy (including such treatments as heat, ultrasound, and massage) may relieve discomfort from cervical and lumbosacral osteoarthritis
5. Know that hip and knee replacement may relieve signs and symptoms of osteoarthritis and restore independence in older adults
6. Assist with planning a weight reduction program, if recommended
7. Apply traction or a cervical collar to relieve nerve root pressure in the neck, if ordered
8. Encourage daily exercise to maintain maximal range of motion
9. Encourage the patient to use a walker or cane to reduce strain on weight-bearing joints, if necessary

D. Evaluation
   1. The patient experiences relief of pain
   2. The patient maintains maximal joint mobility

XVIII. Osteoporosis

A. General information
   1. Osteoporosis is a bone disorder in which an imbalance between bone formation and resorption leads to bone demineralization
   2. Bones become porous, brittle, and abnormally vulnerable to fracture
   3. Approximately 15 to 20 million Americans have osteoporosis
   4. Osteoporosis may develop insidiously
   5. Osteoporosis is eight times more common in women than in men (women undergo rapid bone loss for 5 years after menopause)
   6. Some degree of osteoporosis is a normal age-related change; the ability to absorb calcium from the intestines decreases with age
   7. Other factors associated with osteoporosis include:
      a. Heredity
      b. Small frame
      c. Inactivity
      d. Estrogen deficiency (in postmenopausal women)
      e. Calcium deficiency
      f. Poor nutritional status
      g. Prolonged corticosteroid administration
      h. Prolonged heparin therapy
      i. Alcoholism
      j. Diabetes mellitus
      k. Cigarette smoking
      l. Rheumatoid arthritis
   8. In advanced osteoporosis, vertebral compression fractures and kyphosis may cause compression of the heart, lungs, and nerves and decrease thoracic mobility; such compression may lead to respiratory and cardiac problems

9. Even minor trauma may cause fractures, especially of the wrist (Colles' fracture), vertebrae (T_{12} and L_1), and hip
10. Fractures caused by osteoporosis pose a serious threat to the older adult's independence

B. Assessment findings
   1. The patient may make such vague complaints as easy fatigability, general arm and leg weakness, headache, and an insecure feeling when walking
   2. Height may decrease over months or years
   3. The patient may have lower dorsal kyphosis ("dowager's hump" or "widow's hump") with abdominal protrusion, from compression fractures of the vertebrae (especially the lower thoracic and lumbar vertebrae)
   4. A rounded back and shortened trunk may make the extremities look disproportionately long
   5. The ribs and iliac crest typically angle downward
   6. Decreased thorax size may cause changes in respiratory function
   7. Limited movement may make bending and stair-climbing difficult
   8. Diagnostic tests help rule out conditions that may masquerade as osteoporosis, such as osteoarthritis
   9. Serum calcium, inorganic phosphorus, and alkaline phosphatase levels are normal in older adults with osteoporosis
   10. X-rays may show degeneration of the lower thoracic and lumbar vertebrae
   11. Bone biopsy reveals thin, porous, but otherwise normal bone

C. Nursing implications
   1. Keep in mind that nursing goals are to slow or halt bone loss, to remineralize bone, and to minimize the risk of falls
   2. Teach the patient how to perform daily activities without carrying heavy objects or making sudden bending or lifting movements
   3. Teach the patient about safety precautions to help prevent falls, such as:
      a. Using nonskid rugs to prevent slipping
      b. Wearing well-fitting low-heeled shoes
      c. Ensuring clear lighting
      d. Keeping pathways unobstructed
   4. Advise the patient to consume a high-calcium diet with adequate fluoride and vitamin D; warn against excessive phosphorus intake
   5. Administer analgesics for pain, as ordered
   6. If estrogen therapy is prescribed, teach the patient about potential side effects; emphasize the importance of close follow-up and ongoing reevaluation
   7. Encourage the patient to engage in an exercise program carefully adjusted for the patient's condition and capability, to help strengthen bones

8. Provide psychological support to help the patient cope with changes in body image and life-style

D. Evaluation
  1. The patient's bone loss is minimized
  2. The patient avoids fractures

XIX. Renal failure

A. General information
  1. Renal failure refers to inability of the kidneys to excrete metabolites; it may be acute or chronic
  2. The incidence of chronic renal failure has increased among older adults
  3. Urinary tract infections and renovascular disease secondary to hypertension are the leading causes of renal failure in older adults
  4. Normal age-related changes in renal function place older adults at higher risk for developing renal failure from any compromise in renal function
  5. Older adults may develop renal failure from neglected, delayed, or inadequate treatment of the following conditions:
    a. Insufficient fluid intake
    b. Fluid loss from diarrhea, vomiting, or hemorrhage
    c. Cardiac failure
    d. Inappropriate use of diuretics and laxatives
    e. Urinary tract infection
    f. Urinary tract obstruction caused by calculi or prostatic hypertrophy
  6. Causes of acute renal failure in older adults include:
    a. Hypotensive episode
    b. Antibiotic overdose
    c. Hypovolemia
  7. Acute renal failure may progress to chronic renal failure
  8. In older adults, chronic renal failure commonly results from other chronic illnesses, such as uncontrolled hypertension and diabetes mellitus; other causes include chronic glomerulonephritis, polycystic kidney disease, and cancer
  9. The prognosis depends on the presence of other organic or systemic diseases and the patient's ability to adapt to disease, therapy, and life-style changes
  10. Common complications of renal failure in older adults include:
    a. Anemia
    b. Renal osteodystrophy
    c. Hypertension
    d. Arrhythmias
    e. CHF
    f. Pericarditis
    g. CNS and peripheral neuropathy

      h. Dry, itchy skin
11. Renal failure affects every body system
12. For older adults with chronic renal failure, three treatment options usually are available:
      a. Conservative treatment (such as food and fluid restrictions and electrolyte replacement therapy), whose goals include preserving remaining renal function, managing any reversible causes of renal failure, and relieving symptoms caused by uremia
      b. Hemodialysis, in which waste products and excess water are removed by circulating blood through a dialyzer
      c. Peritoneal dialysis, in which cleansing fluid is instilled into the peritoneal cavity to remove waste products and fluid by means of osmosis

B. Assessment findings
1. Early detection of renal failure may be difficult because normal age-related changes and various diseases may mask signs and symptoms
2. Initially, hyponatremia may occur; this condition causes hypotension, dry mouth, loss of skin turgor, listlessness, fatigue, and nausea
3. Later signs and symptoms of renal failure include somnolence (sleepiness) and confusion; as the disorder progresses, sodium retention, hyperkalemia, and fluid overload may arise
4. As urine output decreases, urine may become dilute and contain casts and crystals
5. Hypertension may occur from fluid or sodium excess or from excessive renin production
6. CHF may develop from fluid overload
7. Dyspnea and pulmonary congestion may result from CHF
8. Pericardial inflammation may result from uremia
9. Arrhythmias may develop from electrolyte imbalances
10. Kussmaul's respirations may result from acidosis
11. Renal failure increases the risk for the following infections:
      a. Staphylococcal infections of dialysis shunts, fistulae, peritoneal catheters, and open wounds
      b. *Candida albicans,* a common fungal organism affecting the buccal mucosa
         (1) In this infection, white plaques form and may develop into ulcers, which may spread to the esophagus
         (2) Dysphagia may result
12. Dry mouth, metallic taste, and uremic odor may be present
13. Anorexia, nausea, and vomiting may occur
14. GI inflammation and ulcerations may develop
15. Anemia may arise; its severity and signs and symptoms vary
16. Bleeding and clotting disorders occur in late renal failure, with the following clinical manifestations:
      a. Epistaxis

b. Increased occult intestinal blood loss
c. Bruising after trauma
17. Neuropathy results from uremic waste buildup; this disorder is characterized by tingling and restlessness (usually in the lower extremities) and loss of motor strength and grip
18. Headache, lassitude, memory changes, and decreased mental function may develop
19. Skin may appear yellow or sallow
20. Bone demineralization may occur, possibly without symptoms in early stages of the disease
21. In later stages of the disease, clinical features may include:
a. Bone pain
b. Stress fractures
c. Deposits of calcium phosphate crystals in soft tissues of the muscles, joints, and blood vessels
22. The BUN level is elevated above 70 mg/dl
23. The serum creatinine level is elevated (according to age-corrected norms)
24. Uric acid and serum phosphorus levels may be elevated; the serum calcium level may be low
25. Urinalysis may show protein, glucose, erythrocytes, leukocytes, and casts
26. Urine specific gravity may be fixed at 1.010
27. Kidney biopsy may be performed to detect underlying pathologic conditions

C. Nursing implications
1. Keep in mind that nursing goals are to relieve symptoms, to prevent complications, and to help the patient maintain an acceptable quality of life
2. Teach the patient how to plan meals that are low in protein, potassium, and sodium
3. Inform the patient of the importance of following prescribed fluid restrictions
4. Stress the importance of frequent and meticulous mouth care to prevent oral infections
5. Monitor for signs and symptoms of hyperkalemia, including diarrhea and leg and abdominal cramps
6. Monitor for signs and symptoms of fluid overload:
a. Edema
b. Weight gain
c. Hypertension
d. Shortness of breath
e. ORTHOPNEA
f. Crackles

7. Explain the importance of using superfatted soaps, oatmeal baths, and skin lotion to manage pruritus
8. Help the anemic patient cope with a low energy level by restructuring activities and setting priorities for energy expenditure
9. Help the patient follow the multiple-medication regimen by giving careful instructions, reinforcing instructions, and developing reminders to simplify medication administration
10. Monitor for medication side effects and drug interactions
11. Monitor for joint and bone complications; reinforce the importance of safety measures to prevent fractures
12. Be familiar with specific nursing implications of hemodialysis and peritoneal dialysis
13. Foster independence by encouraging the patient to maximize activity and to take part in decision making
14. Provide emotional support for the patient and family
15. When dialysis is poorly tolerated and the patient becomes dependent or mentally incapacitated, support the patient and family in their decision of whether to continue treatment
16. Provide emotional and physical comfort to the patient who terminates treatment

D. Evaluation
1. The patient experiences relief of symptoms
2. The patient successfully adapts to life-style changes related to diet, medication, activity level, and dialysis treatments

XX. Thyrotoxicosis

A. General information
1. Thyrotoxicosis is a disorder caused by excessive thyroid hormone production and its effect on body tissues
2. Disorders most frequently associated with thyrotoxicosis include:
   a. Graves' disease
   b. Toxic nodular goiter
   c. Subacute thyroiditis
3. The cause of thyrotoxicosis is unknown; autoimmune, psychological, traumatic, and hereditary factors are suspected
4. In older adults, thyrotoxicosis may precipitate CHF, acute pulmonary edema, and angina
5. Thyrotoxic crisis (thyroid storm) is an acute manifestation of thyrotoxicosis that may occur in persons with preexisting (and perhaps unrecognized) disease; it is precipitated by a stressful event (such as trauma, surgery, or infection) and may be fatal if untreated

B. Assessment findings
1. In older adults, signs and symptoms of thyrotoxicosis may be absent or mistaken for those of more common diseases

2. Signs and symptoms of thyrotoxicosis include:
   a. Nervousness
   b. Tremor
   c. Weight loss
   d. Heat intolerance with excessive perspiration
   e. Emotional lability
   f. Proximal muscle weakness
   g. Diarrhea
   h. Tachycardia
   i. Widened pulse pressure
   j. Warm, smooth skin
   k. Thyroid enlargement or abnormality
   l. EXOPHTHALMOS (less common in older adults)
3. Weight loss and CHF may be the primary signs of thyrotoxicosis in older adults
4. Other common clinical features of thyrotoxicosis in older adults include:
   a. Nervousness
   b. Fine tremors
   c. Weight loss despite an excellent appetite
   d. Tachycardia not relieved by sleep or rest
5. Thyrotoxic crisis has an abrupt onset and may cause such signs and symptoms as:
   a. Tachycardia
   b. Irritability
   c. Hyperkinesia
   d. High fever
   e. Visual disturbances
   f. Vomiting
   g. Diarrhea
   h. Hypertension
6. An elevated level of serum protein-bound iodine reflects increased thyroid activity, which may result in excessive thyroid hormone secretion
7. Radioimmunoassay shows increased serum T_4 and T_3 concentrations
8. A TRH stimulation test shows failure of TSH levels to rise within 30 minutes after TRH administration

C. Nursing implications
   1. Keep in mind that nursing goals are to help restore euthyroidism and to provide support and comfort to the patient
   2. Know that primary treatments for thyrotoxicosis include antithyroid drugs, ^{131}I, and surgery
   3. Monitor the patient's vital signs, level of consciousness, serum electrolyte levels, cardiac function, and urinary output
   4. Emphasize the importance of bed rest

5. Provide a quiet, dark, comfortable environment with minimal stimulation to promote rest
6. Be familiar with nursing implications specific to the patient's therapeutic regimen
7. Stay alert for signs and symptoms of thyrotoxic crisis
8. Provide eye care to the patient with exophthalmos or ophthalmopathy by moistening the conjunctivae with isotonic eye drops and advising the patient to wear eyeglasses or eye patches to protect the eyes
9. Teach the patient about the importance of a nutritious, high-calorie diet and vitamin supplements
10. Expect to administer sedatives to promote rest
11. Counsel the patient and family about the course of the disease and inform the family that the patient may show emotional lability at times
12. Emphasize the importance of a quiet, nonstimulating environment
13. Stress the importance of regular medical follow-up care

D. Evaluation
1. The patient regains and maintains euthyroidism
2. The patient avoids complications

XXI. Urinary tract infection

A. General information
1. Urinary tract infection (UTI) refers to the presence of microorganisms in the urinary tract, including the bladder, urethra, prostate, or kidneys
2. The incidence of UTI increases with age
3. Patients with debilitating or chronic illness are at high risk for UTI and potentially severe complications
4. UTI is more common in women than men because the female's urethra is shorter than the male's
5. Older adult men are at higher risk for developing UTI than younger men because of prostatic hypertrophy
6. UTI usually results from *Escherichia coli* or other gram-negative enteric bacteria
7. Risk factors for UTI include:
   a. Urinary stasis, retention, and obstruction
   b. Institutionalization (such as in a hospital or nursing home), which increases exposure to bacteria
   c. Diabetes mellitus
   d. Renal failure
   e. Hypertension
   f. CVA
   g. Dementia
   h. Sexual activity
   i. Use of catheters or other instrumentation

8. Conditions that predispose older adults to urinary stasis, retention, and obstruction include:
   a. Urethral or ureteral stenosis
   b. Urethral or ureteral strictures
   c. Renal calculi
   d. Immobility
   e. Tumors
   f. Neurologic changes resulting from CVA
   g. CYSTOCELE (in women)
   h. Prostatic hypertrophy (in men)
9. If untreated, UTI may progress to bacteremia or renal failure
10. The decision of whether to treat asymptomatic bacteriuria in older adults varies among physicians

B. Assessment findings
   1. Older adults with UTI may be asymptomatic or exhibit only vague signs and symptoms
   2. Signs and symptoms of UTI include:
      a. Lower abdominal discomfort
      b. Urinary frequency
      c. Urinary urgency
      d. Dysuria
      e. Nocturia
      f. Turbid urine
      g. Fever
      h. Chills
      i. Hematuria
      j. Vomiting
   3. The diagnosis of UTI is confirmed by a quantitative urine culture revealing a bacterial count of 100,000/ml or more
   4. Gram stain identifies the specific bacteria present
   5. A follow-up urine culture is done after 10 days to determine the effectiveness of antibiotic therapy

C. Nursing implications
   1. Keep in mind that the nursing goal is to resolve UTI and prevent its recurrence
   2. Explain to the patient the importance of maintaining adequate fluid intake (2,500 to 3,000 ml/24 hours)
   3. Verify urine cultures, causative organism, drug sensitivity, and drug allergies before initiating prescribed antibiotic therapy
   4. Stress the importance of strict compliance with the antibiotic therapeutic regimen
   5. Teach the patient about potential antibiotic side effects
   6. Provide the patient with a written schedule for antibiotic therapy, including specific instructions (for instance, "Take 1 hour before or after meals")

7. Teach the sexually active older adult how to prevent UTI through such methods as:
    a. Bathing before and after intercourse
    b. Voiding immediately after intercourse
    c. Using alternative intercourse positions to reduce stress placed on the woman's urethra by the male-superior position
8. Teach the patient how to perform perineal hygiene (cleansing the perineum from front to back) to prevent fecal bacteria from entering the urethra
9. Inform the patient who is prone to UTI about the possible benefits of a diet that promotes acidic urine to prevent growth of pathogens; appropriate foods include prunes, plums, cranberries, grains, meats, eggs, cheese, and fish
10. Promote periodic activity and meticulous perineal care for the patient with limited mobility
11. Suspect and investigate for UTI in a patient whose voiding habits have changed
12. Teach the patient the purpose of medications used to prevent UTI or decrease its frequency, such as methenamine salts (Mandelamine, Hiprex) and nitrofurantoin (Furadantin, Macrodantin)
13. Instruct the patient to avoid irritating chemicals, such as harsh soaps, powders, bubble baths, and deodorants, when cleansing the perineal area because these products may alter perineal pH and impair tissue integrity
14. Teach the patient to avoid caffeine, which may irritate the bladder
15. Recommend warm sitz baths to help relieve discomfort
16. Warn the patient receiving phenazopyridine, a urinary analgesic, that this drug may turn urine red-orange
17. Advise the patient to urinate at the first urge
18. Suggest that a female patient wear pantyhose with a ventilated cotton crotch and cotton (rather than synthetic-fiber) underpants to allow perineal ventilation and absorption of vaginal discharge
19. Follow proper aseptic technique during insertion of a urinary indwelling catheter
20. Maintain a sterile closed system when using a urinary drainage system
21. Be aware of the major entry points for bacteria in a urinary drainage system:
    a. Urethral meatus
    b. Junction between the catheter and collection tube
    c. Connection to the drainage bag
    d. Open end of the drainage spigot
22. Position the drainage bag below bladder level and off the floor
23. Teach the patient and family about proper care and maintenance of the indwelling catheter

D. Evaluation
   1. The patient's UTI resolves
   2. The patient avoids UTI recurrences
   3. The patient's indwelling catheter is managed properly

XXII. Venous insufficiency

A. General information
   1. Venous insufficiency refers to an interference with venous blood flow, resulting in compromised circulation to the tissues
      a. The vessels lose their elasticity, causing varicosities (elongated and dilated)
      b. Vessels occlude and may rupture
      c. Efficiency of valves is reduced
   2. Varicosity, venous thrombosis, and chronic venous insufficiency from valvular destruction are associated with age-related vascular changes, all of which interfere with venous blood flow
   3. Varicosity usually affects superficial veins, such as the greater and lesser saphenous veins
      a. Varicose veins result from structural changes in the venous walls and valves, leading to pooling of blood and edema; veins become increasingly dilated, tortuous, and serpentine
      b. Older adults with varicose veins are at high risk for venous thrombosis
   4. The increased incidence of venous thrombosis in older adults is associated with progressive enlargement of intramuscular calf veins, which occurs with aging
      a. Deep-vein thrombosis is a serious condition that increases the risk of pulmonary embolism; it involves calf veins, including the peroneal and posterior tibial veins
      b. Superficial venous thrombosis typically involves the greater and lesser saphenous veins; it usually is self-limiting
   5. Precipitating factors for venous thrombosis include:
      a. Stress causing injury to the vessel intima
      b. Altered blood coagulability
      c. Blood stasis
      d. Fractures
      e. Immobility
      f. Surgery
      g. Obesity
      h. Debilitating diseases and disorders, such as CHF, neoplasm, chronic infection, and CVA
   6. Bed rest increases the risk of venous thrombosis in older adults
   7. Venous thrombosis rarely develops without associated inflammation; in thrombophlebitis, both a thrombus and inflammation are present

B. Assessment findings
  1. Varicose veins may appear swollen, distended, and knotted and usually are located in subcutaneous leg tissues
  2. Varicosities develop gradually and may cause mild to severe symptoms or no symptoms at all
  3. Signs and symptoms of varicose veins include:
    a. Feeling of heaviness in the legs
    b. Leg cramps at night
    c. Diffuse, dull, aching pain after standing or walking
    d. Easy fatigue
    e. Palpable nodules
  4. In advanced stages, varicose veins may become thick and hard to the touch and cause dull or stabbing pain; impaired circulation may cause ulcers in the lower part of the legs
  5. Signs and symptoms of chronic venous insufficiency include:
    a. Chronic leg edema
    b. Tissue fibrosis and induration
    c. Skin discoloration from blood extravasation in subcutaneous tissues
    d. Stasis ulcers
  6. Signs and symptoms of thrombophlebitis include:
    a. Tenderness, redness, and warmth over a hard, stringlike vein
    b. Homan's sign (calf pain with dorsiflexion of the foot)
    c. Edema in the affected extremity
  7. Diagnostic tests to detect venous thrombosis include:
    a. Contrast venography
    b. Doppler ultrasonography
    c. Radioactive-labeled fibrinogen
    d. Impedance plethysmography
    e. Phlebography

C. Nursing implications
  1. Keep in mind that nursing goals for the patient with venous insufficiency are to promote comfort, to minimize varicosities, and to prevent formation of thrombi and emboli
  2. Caution the patient with varicose veins not to wear constrictive clothing
  3. Suggest that the patient wear antiembolism stockings to promote venous return; stockings should be worn from the proximal foot to just below the knee and should be applied after elevating the leg for 5 minutes to prevent blood trapping
  4. Encourage the patient to elevate the legs for 1 to 2 hours periodically during the day
  5. Advise the patient to avoid prolonged standing
  6. Encourage the patient to walk regularly to prevent venous stasis
  7. Teach the patient to stay alert for thrombophlebitis and stasis ulcers

8. Be familiar with the nursing implications of specific medications and surgical treatments
9. Know that nursing interventions for thrombophlebitis may include:
   a. Enforcing bed rest for 4 to 10 days, as prescribed
   b. Elevating the patient's leg to decrease pain, edema, and venous stasis
   c. Instructing the patient to wear elastic stockings while in bed and always to wear such stockings when ambulating (to compress veins and promote venous return)
   d. Teaching the patient to avoid prolonged sitting or standing
   e. Applying warm moist packs to the entire length of the affected extremity to relieve vasospasm and inflammation
   f. Administering anticoagulation therapy or fibrinolytic medication, as ordered
10. Stay alert for signs and symptoms of pulmonary embolism, such as dyspnea, chest pain, and tachycardia; if pulmonary embolism is suspected, notify the physician at once

D. Evaluation
   1. The patient experiences relief of symptoms
   2. The patient avoids complications
   3. The patient avoids stasis ulcers

Points to remember

In older adults, signs and symptoms of some pathologic health problems may be subtle and variable, and commonly differ from those seen in younger persons.

Cataracts are among the most common eye problems in older adults.

COPD is the major cause of respiratory disability in older adults.

Immobility is the single biggest risk factor for development of decubitus ulcers.

The most common forms of dementia are multi-infarct dementia and Alzheimer's disease.

Glucose intolerance among older adults may result from age-related changes in insulin levels, insulin release, reduced peripheral effectiveness of insulin, or a combination of these factors.

Normal age-related changes place older adults at higher risk for renal failure from any compromise in renal function.

Glossary

The following terms are defined in Appendix A, page 194.

aphasia	dysarthria
apraxia	dysphagia
arteriosclerosis obliterans	dysphasia
astereognosis	eschar
claudication	exophthalmos
crepitus	hemianopia
cystocele	hemiplegia
delirium	homonymous hemianopia
dementia	hyperemia
diplopia	hypertonia

Glossary *(continued)*

hyphema

ischemia

miotic

mydriatic

orthopnea

paraphasia

paresis

paresthesia

phacoemulsification

polydipsia

polyphagia

polyuria

proprioception

pulse pressure

stenosis

uveitis

Valsalva maneuver

Study questions

To evaluate your understanding of this chapter, answer the following questions in the space provided; then compare your responses with the correct answers in Appendix B, pages 202 to 204.

1. What is the nursing goal for the patient with delirium? _____

_____

2. In an older adult who develops an ulcer from chronic arterial insufficiency, the nurse should assess for which clinical features? _____

_____

3. Why are arrhythmias more serious in older adults than in younger adults?

_____

_____

4. Which signs and symptoms should the nurse expect in a patient with cataracts? _____

_____

5. In a patient with left hemiplegia secondary to CVA, the nurse should expect which assessment findings related to speech? _____

_____

6. What are the nursing goals for an older adult with CHF? _____

_____

7. What are three factors that place older adults at increased risk for decubitus ulcers? _____

_____

8. Why is the urine glucose level a poor indicator of blood glucose elevation in older adults? _____

_____

Study questions (continued)

9. Which problems may occur in older adults who consume a high-fiber diet to help manage diverticular disease? _____

_____

10. What are the most common fracture sites in older adults? _____

_____

11. What is the nursing goal for older adults with glaucoma? _____

_____

12. What are three age-related changes that contribute to hypertension in older adults? _____

_____

13. Why is hypothyroidism sometimes hard to detect in older adults? _____

_____

_____

14. What are three common complications of MI in older adults? _____

_____

_____

15. In what part of the body should the nurse expect to find Heberden nodes in a patient with osteoarthritis? _____

_____

16. What are common fracture sites in older adults with osteoporosis? _____

_____

_____

17. What are the leading causes of renal impairment in older adults? _____

_____

_____

Study questions *(continued)*

18. Which signs of thyrotoxicosis may predominate in older adults? _____

_____

_____

19. Which conditions predispose older adults to urinary stasis, retention, and obstruction? _____

_____

20. Which blood vessels are involved in deep-vein thrombosis? _____

_____

_____

CHAPTER 6

Functional Health Problems

Learning objectives

Check off the following items once you've mastered them:

☐ Describe a functional assessment.

☐ Define sensory deprivation.

☐ Identify assessment findings that indicate impaired function in each of the following areas: hearing, vision, taste and smell, and integument.

☐ Identify assessment findings associated with impaired mobility.

☐ Identify assessment findings associated with urinary incontinence.

☐ Describe two nursing interventions for each of the following functional problems: sensory deprivation, auditory impairment, visual impairment, taste and smell alteration, integumentary impairment, mobility impairment, and urinary incontinence.

I. Functional assessment

A. General information
   1. FUNCTIONAL ASSESSMENT is a type of assessment the nurse can use to evaluate an older adult's overall well-being and self-care abilities
   2. Functional assessment findings have multiple uses
      a. They identify individual patient needs and care deficits
      b. They provide the basis for developing a care plan that preserves and enhances the abilities of the older adult with coexisting disease and chronic illness
      c. They help the nurse identify and match the older adult's needs with such services as housekeeping, home health care, and day care to help the patient maintain independence
      d. They provide feedback regarding treatment and rehabilitation
   3. Functional assessment tools must be evaluated for reliability and validity

B. Types of functional assessment
   1. Assessment of *activities of daily living* (ADLs) evaluates the patient's ability to perform daily personal care activities, such as feeding, bathing, toileting, and dressing
   2. Assessment of *instrumental ADLs* evaluates the patient's ability to perform more complex personal care activities, such as cooking, cleaning, and shopping

C. Functional assessment tools
   1. The PULSES (*P*hysical condition, *U*pper limbs, *L*ower limbs, *S*ocial factors, *S*ensory component) profile measures the patient's level of independence and dependence in performing ADLs
   2. The Barthel Index and Barthel Self-Care Rating measures the patient's physical dependence in performing personal care
   3. The FANCAPES (*F*luid, *A*eration, *N*utrition, *C*ommunication, *A*ctivity, *P*ain, *E*limination, *S*ocialization) assessment evaluates the patient's ability to meet personal needs and the extent to which the patient requires assistance
   4. The OARS (*O*lder *A*dult *R*esource *S*ervices) multidimensional functional assessment evaluates the level at which the patient can function; it assesses functional capabilities in such areas as social resources, economic resources, physical health, mental health, and ADLs (see *Key areas of OARS multidimensional functional assessment*, page 112)
   5. The Minimum Data Set for Nursing Home Resident Assessment and Care Screening (MDS) is a standardized tool used in Medicare/Medicaid nursing homes to assess a patient's physical, mental, and psychosocial functioning

KEY AREAS OF O.A.R.S. MULTIDIMENSIONAL FUNCTIONAL ASSESSMENT

The OARS multidimensional functional assessment is divided into two parts. Part A addresses the individual's level of functioning. Part B addresses the individual's use of resources. The chart below highlights the type of assessment data collected for Parts A and B.

PART A	
SECTION	TYPE OF ASSESSMENT DATA
Demographics	• Address • Date • Interviewee or informant • Place of interview • Duration of interview • Sex • Race • Age • Education • Telephone number
Social resources	• Marital status • Resident companions • Extent and type of contact with others • Availability of confidante • Perception of loneliness • Availability, duration, and source of help
Economic resources	• Employee status • Major occupation of self and spouse • Source and amount of income • Number of dependents • Home ownership or rental • Source and adequacy of financial resources • Health insurance • Subjective interpretation of income adequacy
Mental health	• Short Portable Mental Status Questionnaire (SPMSQ) test of organicity (level of orientation, remote and recent memory, practical skills, and basic mathematical ability, such as serial subtraction) • Extent of worry, satisfaction, and interest in life • Present mental status and change in past years • Short Psychiatric Evaluation schedule (15-item evaluation)
Physical health	• Physician visits, days sick, hospitalized (in hospital or nursing home) in past 6 months • Medications • Current illness and extent of interference • Physical, visual, and hearing disabilities • Alcoholism • Participation in exercise • Self-assessment of health

(continued)

```
┌────────────────────────────────────────────────────────────────┐
│ KEY AREAS OF O.A.R.S. MULTIDIMENSIONAL FUNCTIONAL                │
│ ASSESSMENT (continued)                                           │
└────────────────────────────────────────────────────────────────┘
```

PART B

SECTION	TYPE OF ASSESSMENT DATA
Services	• Transportation • Social and recreation services • Remedial training • Mental health • Psychotropic drugs • Personal care • Nursing care • Medical care • Physical therapy • Continuous supervision • Checking • Relocation and placement services • Homemaker • Meal preparation • Financial assistance • Coordination, information, and referral

From Fillenbaum, G.G. "Multidimensional Functional Assessment of Older Adults." The Duke Older Americans Resources and Services. Erlbaum, Hillsdale, N.J. 1988. Adapted with permission of the publisher.

II. Sensory deprivation

A. General information
1. Sensory deprivation is characterized by:
   a. Decrease in sensory input
   b. Decrease in meaningful activity or in relevance of stimuli
   c. Alteration in the RETICULAR ACTIVATING SYSTEM
2. In older adults, sensory impairments are cumulative, occur over time, compound each other, and may lead to or potentiate sensory deprivation
3. Sensory deprivation, sensory distortion, and sensory overload may coexist in older adults
4. Older adults are especially vulnerable to misperception or decreased perception of sensory stimuli from the following factors:
   a. Physiologic changes associated with aging or illness that interfere with perception or reception of stimuli
   b. Structural features of the environment or treatment forms that distort, disrupt, make monotonous, mute, intensify, or disorganize stimuli in a way that destroys the order and meaning of stimuli

      c. Caregiver expectations of appropriate behavior (as manifested by staff members prohibiting or discouraging patient behaviors that promote interpretation of stimuli, such as exploration and verbal communication)

  5. Acute health problems (such as dehydration, high fever, and shock) may cause sensory alterations in older adults, making them vulnerable to sensory deprivation

  6. Social isolation is a major component of sensory deprivation in older adults

  7. Sensory deprivation may be mislabeled or overlooked in older adults because its manifestations resemble those associated with senility

B. Assessment findings
  1. Responses to sensory deprivation vary from one person to the next
  2. Cognitive function changes caused by sensory deprivation may include:
    a. Confusion
    b. Disorientation
    c. General slowing of intellectual activity
    d. Difficulty with concentration and abstract thinking
    e. Impaired problem solving
    f. Inability to think coherently
  3. Emotional responses to sensory deprivation may include:
    a. Anxiety
    b. Fear
    c. Depression
    d. Rapid mood swings
  4. Perceptual changes caused by sensory deprivation may be visual, auditory, kinesthetic, or somatesthetic and may vary from mild daydreams to illusions and hallucinations
  5. Behavioral changes caused by sensory deprivation may include:
    a. Noncompliant behavior
    b. Wandering
    c. Purposeless activity

C. Nursing implications
  1. Keep in mind that the nursing goal is to promote an optimal level of sensory input
  2. Be aware that sensory deprivation results from a combination of physiologic, psychological, and environmental factors
  3. Maximize the patient's remaining sensory functions by correcting deficits to help reduce sensory deprivation; for instance, help the patient obtain eyeglasses and hearing aids
  4. Use touch to help orient the patient and provide stimulation
  5. Provide all the cues the patient needs to maintain orientation and a sense of reality, such as clocks, calendars, and a predictable daily routine
  6. Encourage the patient to participate in activities according to ability

7. Be aware that background entertainment, such as a television or radio, may interfere with communication
8. Let the patient control the stimulation level
9. Allow the patient to gain knowledge and awareness of the environment by exploring, handling, touching, verbalizing, and asking questions
10. Provide opportunities for the patient to solve problems and make independent decisions; help ensure that problem solving is successful and meaningful
11. Promote interaction between the patient and others
12. Provide goal-directed, focused conversations on topics meaningful to the patient

III. Hearing loss

A. General information
1. Hearing loss is the most common sensory loss experienced by older adults
2. A person with a hearing loss experiences a distortion in sound
3. Sound distortion affects a person's interpretation of the world, possibly leading to social isolation, depression, paranoia, suspiciousness, and impaired problem-solving ability because information cannot be heard
4. Approximately 30% of older adults have hearing loss
   a. Twice as many men as women have hearing loss
   b. About 13% of persons with hearing loss need professional assistance to cope with the problem
5. Auditory changes occur subtly over time
6. SENSORINEURAL HEARING LOSS is a dysfunction in transmission of sound to the brain
   a. Aging typically is accompanied by a progressive, bilaterally symmetrical sensorineural hearing loss (presbycusis)
   b. Presbycusis affects the ability to hear high-pitched sounds and sibilant consonants (such as f, s, th, ch, and sh)
      (1) As hearing loss progresses, perception of the consonants b, t, p, k, and d also is impaired
      (2) Clear perception of consonants is important in understanding language with high-pitched sounds
   c. Excessive cerumen in the middle ear intensifies presbycusis
   d. Background noise may worsen hearing impairment in older adults with presbycusis
7. CONDUCTIVE HEARING LOSS results from an impediment in mechanical transmission of sound along the auditory pathway; the condition may improve with medical treatment or a hearing aid
8. *Mixed hearing loss* refers to a combination of conductive and sensorineural hearing loss

B. Assessment findings
  1. Detection of hearing loss may be difficult because some people adapt to hearing loss over time
  2. Subtle signs of hearing loss include inappropriate responses to questions and failure to respond to questions
  3. Impaired hearing may cause difficulty following verbal directions
  4. The patient may withdraw from social conversations and make frequent requests for clarification and repetition
  5. Other signs of hearing loss include turning of one ear to the speaker while watching the speaker intently and speech with an unusual quality and poor articulation (such as speech that is too loud, too soft, monotonous, or harsh)
  6. With conductive hearing loss, impaired hearing sensitivity usually is the same for all frequencies; speech discrimination may remain unimpaired if speech is loud enough
  7. With sensorineural hearing loss, the patient has trouble understanding speech even when it is loud enough to be heard

C. Nursing implications
  1. Keep in mind that the nursing goal is to maximize the patient's auditory function
  2. Determine the extent of the patient's hearing loss by performing an audiologic examination; complete assessment and evaluation are essential to determining appropriate treatment
  3. Modify communication to help the patient understand speech by using the following techniques:
     a. Face the patient
     b. Get the patient's attention through touch or eye contact
     c. Sit or stand so that the patient can see your lips
     d. Speak slowly and distinctly
     e. Speak in a voice loud enough to be heard without shouting
     f. Use short phrases
     g. Use appropriate body language
     h. Eliminate as much background noise as possible
     i. Use a speaking tube or hearing horn (if the patient has a severe hearing impairment)
  4. Encourage the patient to try a hearing aid (which many older adults require); be aware that the hearing aid must be designed for the patient's specific needs and type of hearing loss
  5. Inform the patient that it will take time to adjust to wearing the hearing aid and to learn how to use and care for it
  6. Stress that the patient will need to change established compensatory patterns (such as asking people to repeat what they have said or not paying attention to conversational cues) to reduce social isolation

7. Suggest that the patient use auditory aids to foster independence, including amplifiers on telephone receivers and telephone bells; lighted telephones signals; and auxiliary speakers for radios, televisions, and tape recorders
8. Post a note at the main nursing station intercom stating that the patient is deaf or hearing impaired
9. During patient teaching sessions, ask the patient to repeat learning points to ensure that content was heard
10. Be aware that many older adults with impaired hearing are ignored or presumed to be senile; nursing can play a major advocacy role in promoting assessment and evaluation for auditory impairment

IV. Visual impairment

A. General information
1. Age-related physiologic changes in the eye may lead to:
   a. Senile MIOSIS
   b. Increased lens opacity, or cataract
   c. Reduced peripheral vision
   d. Yellowing of the lens
   e. Reduced ability to accommodate (presbyopia), which usually leads to hyperopia (farsightedness)
2. With age, breakdown of rhodopsin (visual purple) in response to light rays decreases, contributing to poor adaptation to darkness
3. Macular degeneration, another condition affecting older adults, results from hardening and obstruction of retinal arteries; it causes loss of central vision but leaves peripheral vision unimpaired
4. Diabetic retinopathy is a condition characterized by formation of microaneurysms and small hemorrhages in or on the retina, resulting in vision loss; the condition is progressive, and risk increases with age
5. Glaucoma, a condition characterized by increased intraocular pressure, may damage the optic nerve and lead to blindness; its onset may be acute or gradual
6. Vision loss in older adults increases susceptibility to illusions, withdrawal, disorientation, and social isolation

B. Assessment findings
1. The patient may have difficulty with color perception of blue, violet, and green shades
2. Vision may be impaired in dim light
3. Panoramic vision may be impaired
4. The patient with decreased accommodation may hold objects at a distance to focus on them properly
5. The patient with glaucoma may complain of eye strain and morning headaches that disappear after rising; tonometry examination reveals increased intraocular pressure

6. The patient with cataracts may complain of poor vision, eye fatigue, headaches, increased light sensitivity, and blurred vision or multiple images
7. The patient with macular degeneration may complain that central vision is dark or distorted

C. Nursing implications
1. Keep in mind that the nursing goal is to maximize the patient's visual function
2. Help the patient develop compensatory skills
3. Help the patient with macular degeneration maximize use of peripheral vision
4. Support the postoperative cataract patient in adjusting to distorted vision and using eyeglasses or contact lenses
5. Know that rehabilitation plans should maximize use of nonvisual aids
6. Suggest that the patient use visual aids to foster independence, such as:
   a. Large-print books and magazines
   b. Audiotapes of recorded books
   c. Magnifying glass
   d. Plastic-page device that magnifies a printed page
   e. Large-number push-button telephone
7. Be aware that associations for the blind and other community programs can assist the patient with traveling and obtaining audiotapes
8. Assess the patient's ability to perform ADLs; assist with environmental changes needed to promote independent living
9. Provide support to the patient who recently became blind or who has a visual impairment that causes alterations in self-image, self-esteem, and confidence to function independently

V. Alterations in taste and smell

A. General information
1. The number of taste buds per papilla (elevations covering the tongue surface) decreases with age
2. Taste buds that distinguish sweet and salty flavors show the greatest decline with age
3. Ability to taste is associated with ability to smell
4. Loss of taste and smell directly affects dietary intake and food enjoyment
5. Smoking and dental status affect ability to taste
6. Ability to smell begins to decline at about age 45
7. With decline of smell, older adults may not detect smoke

B. Assessment findings
1. The patient may season food heavily with salt or strong spices to compensate for taste loss

2. The patient may add extra sugar to coffee or tea and may prefer excessively sweet or salty foods

C. Nursing implications
   1. Keep in mind that the nursing goal is to maximize the patient's taste and smell function
   2. Teach the patient about age-related changes in taste and smell
   3. Instruct the patient to use substitutes for salt and sugar, such as spices and seasoning, as indicated by the patient's medical history
   4. Encourage use of smoke detectors to alert the patient to fire

VI. Impaired integument

A. General information
   1. Aging causes generalized thinning of the skin
   2. Aging also leads to dry skin from decreased sebaceous gland activity, thinning of the epidermal layer, and poor fluid intake
      a. Older adults are predisposed to dry skin by environmental elements, decreased humidity, harsh soaps, frequent bathing, and nutritional deficiencies
      b. Itching (pruritus) from dry skin threatens skin integrity (however, other causes of itching, such as scabies, pediculosis, and intertrigo, should be ruled out)
   3. Skin turgor decreases with age, resulting in stiffer, less pliable skin
   4. Wound healing slows with age

B. Assessment findings
   1. Rough, scaly, flaking skin may appear on the patient's face, neck, hands, forearms, sides of the lower trunk, and exterior and lateral aspects of the thighs
   2. Itching may signal dry skin; skin irritation or scratch marks may be visible
   3. Dry skin and itching typically are exacerbated by cold, dry, wintry weather; exposure to sun and wind; and irritating fabrics, such as wool
   4. Skin may bruise easily; hemorrhages known as senile purpura may appear

C. Nursing implications
   1. Keep in mind that nursing goals are to maintain integumentary function and to prevent skin breakdown
   2. Use superfatted soaps to restore a protective lipid film to the patient's skin surface
   3. Incorporate bath oils and other hydrophobic preparations into the patient's bathing routine
   4. Apply lotions or emollients to the patient's skin to help lubricate and hydrate the epidermal layer
   5. Maintain adequate humidity in the patient's environment

6. Advise the patient to avoid irritating clothes and hot showers and baths and to limit the number of baths and showers
7. Advise the patient to maintain an adequate fluid intake

VII. Impaired mobility

A. General information
1. Impaired mobility is a serious problem for older adults
2. Conditions that commonly limit mobility include paresthesia, arthritis, neuromotor disturbances, fractures, energy-depleting illness, poor vision, cerebrovascular accident (stroke), joint or foot pain, angina, and peripheral vascular disease
3. Mobility can be maintained into old age by consistent use of muscles and bones
4. Foot problems can severely limit mobility
5. Complications associated with bed rest and lack of mobility include:
    a. Muscle atrophy
    b. Contractures
    c. Osteoporosis
    d. Decubitus ulcers
    e. Orthostatic hypotension
    f. Urinary calculi
    g. Dehydration
    h. Thromboemboli and pulmonary emboli
    i. Poor appetite
    j. Constipation
    k. Fatigue
    l. Insomnia
    m. Stress
    n. Depression
6. Gait disturbances that develop in older adults can impair mobility
7. Impaired mobility increases the risk of injury and falls
8. Mobility may be restricted from poor-fitting shoes; lack of assistive devices, such as canes and walkers; and fear of falling

B. Assessment findings
1. Gait disturbance and joint deformity or asymmetry are the two most common assessment findings in older adults with impaired mobility
2. Other common findings include:
    a. Decreased range of motion
    b. Joint or extremity pain
    c. Diminished muscle strength
    d. Medically prescribed restrictive treatments, such as casts, splints, and restraints

C. Nursing implications
   1. Keep in mind that nursing goals are to maximize the patient's mobility and to prevent falls; many complications associated with immobility are preventable
   2. Urge the patient to use appropriate ambulatory aids to foster independence; such aids include:
       a. Walkers, including wheeled walkers and walkers with seats
       b. Canes, including tripod canes
       c. Wheelchairs, including motorized wheelchairs
       d. Lifter chairs
   3. Teach the patient about the benefits of exercise and activity
   4. Encourage the patient to engage in a systematic, physician-approved exercise program tailored to individual abilities
   5. Assist and encourage the patient confined to a wheelchair or bed to engage in a modified exercise program
   6. Perform passive range-of-motion exercises for the bedridden patient to prevent contractures and keep joints straight
   7. Assist the bedridden patient in performing active exercises to prevent muscle atrophy
   8. Avoid flexion postures to prevent knee and hip contractures when positioning the bedridden patient
   9. Ensure that the patient confined to a chair or wheelchair receives range-of-motion exercises to prevent knee and hip contractures that may result from sitting all day
  10. Teach the patient the importance of foot care and well-fitting shoes
  11. Promote compliance in the patient receiving physical therapy after a hip fracture or prolonged bed rest
  12. Teach the patient about appropriate safety measures to prevent injury and falls

VIII. Urinary incontinence

A. General information
   1. Urinary incontinence is the inability to control urine passage voluntarily
   2. Urinary incontinence may take various forms
       a. STRESS INCONTINENCE is characterized by weakness of supporting pelvic muscles that renders the bladder outlet incompetent
          (1) The disorder affects mainly women
          (2) It typically occurs during sneezing, coughing, or laughing
       b. OVERFLOW INCONTINENCE is characterized by urine overflow resulting from an obstructive lesion or drug-induced urine retention
          (1) In women, the disorder is associated with obstructive problems, such as trigonitis associated with atrophic vaginitis
          (2) In men, it is associated with prostate problems

     c. NEUROGENIC INCONTINENCE is characterized by alteration in the sensory and motor tracts involved in bladder muscle function

     d. URGENCY INCONTINENCE is characterized by a sudden urge to void followed by passage of large amounts of urine

  3. Urinary incontinence may result from drug use

     a. Diuretics may cause incontinence

     b. Sleeping medications and tranquilizers may cause nighttime incontinence because they depress the neurologic sensation that signals the need to urinate

     c. Drugs that cause urine retention (such as anticholinergic agents and central nervous system depressants) may lead to infection and overflow incontinence

  4. Urinary incontinence may result from problems with toileting (such as generalized weakness) or from difficulty walking to the bathroom, manipulating clothing, or handling the bedpan or urinal

  5. Urinary incontinence affects self-esteem, confidence, and independence and may cause dependence, shame, guilt, and fear

B. Assessment findings

  1. A woman may complain of signs and symptoms of stress incontinence, such as involuntary passage of small amounts of urine when coughing, sneezing, or laughing

  2. Dribbling may occur from overflow or an urge to void followed by involuntary urine passage

  3. Urinalysis may reveal infection as the cause of incontinence

  4. A cystometrogram determines the pattern of the bladder's emptying mechanism

     a. It evaluates detrusor muscle function

     b. It assesses the bladder's neuromuscular function

  5. Neurologic tests determine bladder sensation

C. Nursing implications

  1. Keep in mind that the nursing goal is to assist with efforts to improve the patient's urinary continence

  2. Provide frequent opportunities to void if the patient requires assistance with toileting

  3. Modify the patient's environment to promote toileting, such as by relocating furniture or the bedroom, obtaining portable toilet facilities, or installing an elevated toilet seat or grab rails in the bathroom

  4. Use Velcro fasteners to replace cumbersome buttons and hooks on the patient's clothing, if necessary

  5. Administer estrogen to treat atrophic vaginitis, if ordered

  6. Administer antibiotics to treat acute urinary tract infection, if ordered

  7. Assist the patient in planning daily activities and managing incontinence

  8. Initiate scheduled toileting or bladder retraining to avoid episodes of incontinence

a. Provide privacy and warmth for toileting
b. Toilet the patient every 2 hours during the day and every 4 hours at night
c. Progressively lengthen or shorten toileting intervals
d. Carefully time the patient's fluid intake and medication administration

9. If the patient has trouble voiding, discuss techniques to help trigger voiding, such as running water, stroking the inner aspect of the thigh, and using suprapubic tapping

10. Be aware that an indwelling catheter is indicated for patients with severe urinary retention causing recurrent, symptomatic urinary tract infection or hydronephrosis and for patients with skin rashes, ulcers, and wounds that are irritated by contact with urine

11. Teach KEGEL EXERCISES to a female patient with stress incontinence to strengthen pelvic floor muscles
    a. Identify pelvic floor muscles by placing a finger inside the patient's vagina or rectum and having the patient squeeze the finger; inform the patient that these are the same muscles used to hold back gas or a bowel movement
    b. Tell the patient to squeeze the identified muscles for 10 seconds, then relax for 10 seconds; instruct her *not* to contract her stomach, leg, or buttock muscles
    c. Instruct the patient to do these exercises 15 times in the morning, 15 times in the afternoon, and 20 times at night, or to do them for 10 minutes three times a day
    d. Tell the patient to work up to 25 repetitions at a time
    e. Inform the patient that she will notice an improvement in her condition within 2 to 4 weeks if she does the exercises consistently every day

Points to remember

Functional assessment tools can help the nurse match services with patient needs so that the older adult can maintain independence in the community.

Sensory impairments in older adults occur over time and may lead to or potentiate sensory deprivation.

Many complications caused by impaired mobility and physical inactivity can be prevented.

Urinary incontinence lowers self-esteem and confidence and may cause dependence, shame, guilt, and fear.

Glossary

The following terms are defined in Appendix A, page 194.

conductive hearing loss	overflow incontinence
functional assessment	reticular activating system
Kegel exercise	sensorineural hearing loss
miosis	stress incontinence
neurogenic incontinence	urgency incontinence

Study questions

To evaluate your understanding of this chapter, answer the following questions in the space provided; then compare your responses with the correct answers in Appendix B, page 204.

1. What are two types of functional assessment that the nurse can conduct on older adults? _____

2. The nurse should expect which cognitive function changes in a patient with sensory deprivation? _____

3. When caring for a patient with impaired hearing, the nurse can use which techniques to modify communication skills? _____

4. The nurse would observe which action in a patient with poor visual accommodation? _____

5. At what age does the sense of smell begin to decline? _____

6. How does aging affect skin turgor? _____

7. Which conditions commonly limit mobility in older adults? _____

8. What are four types of urinary incontinence? _____

CHAPTER 7

Health Promotion, Safety, and Special Concerns

Learning objectives

Check off the following items once you've mastered them:

☐ Identify major age-related physiologic changes that place older adults at risk for injury from falls.

☐ Name three major factors that contribute to medication problems in older adults.

☐ Describe special exercise precautions that older adults should follow.

☐ Name three factors that contribute to sleep disturbances in older adults.

☐ Identify three common problems with sexual function experienced by older adults.

☐ Name three factors that influence diet and nutrition in older adults.

I. Falls

A. General information
   1. The risk of falls and subsequent complications increases with age
   2. Falls are the second leading cause of accidental death; approximately 75% of falls involve older adults
   3. Women in the old-old age group who live alone are at highest risk for falls
   4. Institutionalized older adults have a higher incidence of falls than do those living in the community; most falls occurring in institutions take place during the evening and night shifts and at change of shifts
   5. Falls contribute to increased hospital stays and increased medical care costs
   6. Many falls result from environmental hazards
   7. Most falls occur at home
   8. Falls commonly lead to fractures of the hip and wrist in older adults
   9. Injuries from falls pose a serious threat to the well-being of older adults, especially those who suffer repeated falls
   10. Immobilization during recovery from a fall increases the risk of complications in older adults

B. Contributing factors
   1. The combination of a weakened skeleton, a weakened support system, and a change in the center of gravity predisposes older adults to falls and other accidents
   2. Mobility hinges on a complex integration of movement, gravity, and equilibrium; with age, this integration may become more difficult, increasing the risk for falls
   3. Falls may result from sudden loss of muscle tone without a specific cause or from loss of consciousness without warning (sometimes called a "drop attack")
   4. Additional physical factors contribute to falls in older adults
      a. Muscle weakness
      b. Gait changes
      c. Decreased sensory awareness
      d. Visual impairment
   5. Certain environmental factors also contribute to falls
      a. Improper footwear
      b. Obstacles in the path
      c. Wet floors
      d. Poor lighting
   6. Cardiovascular diseases that decrease cardiac output or cerebral blood flow also increase the risk of falls
   7. Neurologic disorders causing decreased cerebral blood flow, diminished sensorium, or impaired locomotion may lead to falls

8. Urinary urgency caused by age-related physiologic changes (such as benign prostatic hypertrophy) puts older adults at risk for falling when rushing to the bathroom
9. Falls are associated with use of such medications as diuretics (which cause frequent urination) and hypnotic agents, tranquilizers, sedatives, and pain medications (all of which can cause drowsiness)
10. Older adults who use multiple medications or have multiple medical problems have an increased incidence of falls
11. Altered mental states, such as from stress, depression, confusion, and impaired judgment, may contribute to falls and injury
12. Osteoporosis, which weakens bones, increases the risk of fracture from a fall

C. Nursing implications
1. Keep in mind that nursing goals are to provide appropriate care for fractures and other injuries and to teach the patient how to avoid falls
2. Identify older adults at high risk for falls from advanced age, confusion, unfamiliar surroundings, chronic illness, balance or gait changes, and medications that cause sensory impairment
3. Assess the patient's home for environmental hazards, such as broken stairs, uneven or icy walks, inadequate lighting, frayed carpets, throw rugs, and exposed electric cords
4. Advise the patient to paint stair edges a bright color to increase their visibility
5. Take other measures to make the patient's home safe, such as making sure handrails are present and secured and removing or securing loose carpets and throw rugs
6. Advise the patient to keep outdoor steps and walkways in good repair
7. Instruct the patient to use extra caution when going outside during inclement weather
8. Urge the patient to install handrails in the bathroom and to place nonskid tracks in the bathtub
9. Advise the patient to avoid climbing ladders or using stepstools or chairs to reach objects
10. Instruct the patient to avoid walking on highly polished floors
11. Recommend that the patient use night lights
12. Teach the patient to change position slowly to avoid orthostatic hypotension, which can cause a fall
13. Encourage the patient to wear shoes with adequate support and nonskid heels

II. Hypothermia

A. General information
1. Hypothermia is a condition of below-normal core body temperature: 95° F (35° C) or lower

2. Older adults may suffer accidental hypothermia after exposure to relatively mild cold
3. Older adults who are at increased risk for hypothermia include:
   a. Those with inadequate housing or heating
   b. Those who live alone
   c. Those with a chronic illness
   d. Those who have disorders affecting the ability of vessels to constrict or dilate in response to temperature changes and those who are taking drugs with such vascular effects
4. Hypothermia may exacerbate a preexisting medical condition by depressing body functions
5. Signs and symptoms of hypothermia include:
   a. Pale, waxy skin that is cold to the touch even though the patient is not shivering
   b. Arrhythmias and bradycardia
   c. Hypotension
   d. Muscle rigidity, slurred speech, and drowsiness

B. Contributing factors
   1. Ingestion of substances that accelerate body heat loss, such as alcohol, imipramine, and salicylates, increases the risk of hypothermia
   2. Phenothiazines may impair thermoregulation in older adults
   3. Various factors increase the risk of hypothermia in older adults undergoing surgery
      a. Impaired heat regulation resulting from preoperative medications
      b. Cold temperature in the operating room
      c. Cold solutions
      d. Lack of covering
   4. Older adults may feel comfortably warm even though their bodies are cold; unaware of reduced body temperature, they may not take precautions to prevent hypothermia
   5. Hypoproteinemia may increase the risk of hypothermia in undernourished older adults

C. Nursing implications
   1. Keep in mind that nursing goals are to rewarm the patient slowly and to teach the patient how to prevent hypothermia
   2. If hypothermia is suspected, warm the patient's hands and feet and add covers
   3. If the patient's core temperature drops below 90° F (32.2° C), rewarm the patient slowly under close observation and monitor for arrhythmias and hypokalemia
   4. Do not raise the patient's body temperature more than 1° F (0.6° C) per hour
   5. Do not use electric blankets or hot water bottles because they may cause vasodilation, which may lead to hypotension from inability to maintain cardiac output

6. Measure temperature rectally to assess the patient's core temperature
7. Keep room temperature between 68° and 70° F (20° and 21.1° C) to prevent hypothermia
8. Advise older adults to dress warmly, eat well, and stay as active as possible
9. Teach older adults to wear adequate clothing and to use sufficient blankets to keep warm during sleep
10. Caution older adults about drugs that may affect body temperature
11. For older adults who live alone, suggest that friends or neighbors call or visit once or twice a day, especially during cold weather

III. Hyperthermia

A. General information
1. Hyperthermia has not been defined specifically for older adults; however, usually it is considered to be a core body temperature of 100° F (37.8° C) or higher
2. Common causes of hyperthermia in older adults include infection and an ambient temperature that exceeds body temperature
3. Signs and symptoms vary with the degree of hyperthermia
4. With a core temperature of 100° F, the patient may exhibit:
   a. Apathy
   b. Weakness
   c. Faintness
   d. Headache
5. As core temperature rises above 100° F, the patient may exhibit:
   a. Tachycardia
   b. Weakness
   c. Dry mouth
   d. Increased respirations
   e. Hallucinations
   f. Delusions
   g. Confusion
6. Heat stroke is impaired thermoregulation that results in excessive storage of heat caused by the body's inability to dissipate heat through convection, radiation, and perspiration; heat stroke is characterized by:
   a. Severe tachycardia
   b. Severe tachypnea
   c. Severe frank hypotension
   d. Alteration in consciousness
   e. Rectal temperature of 105° F (40.5° C) or higher
7. Heat syncope may occur in a person who is not acclimated to hot weather; signs and symptoms include:
   a. Dizziness
   b. Fatigue
   c. Sudden faintness after physical exertion

8. Heat exhaustion — less severe than heat stroke — is common in older adults; signs and symptoms include:
   a. Moderate temperature increase (usually no higher than 100° F [37.8° C])
   b. Orthostatic hypotension
   c. Malaise
   d. Irritability
   e. Anxiety
   f. Tachypnea
   g. Tachycardia
   h. Headache
   i. Dizziness
   j. Syncope
9. Central nervous system disturbances and elevated levels of serum glutamic oxaloacetic transaminase, lactate dehydrogenase, and creatinine phosphokinase associated with heat stroke may help distinguish it from heat exhaustion

B. Contributing factors
   1. Various age-related factors increase the risk of hyperthermia
      a. Reduced number of sweat glands, which impairs the body's ability to cool itself
      b. Urinary tract infections
      c. Circulatory problems
      d. Dehydration
   2. Older adults may be unaware of a higher body temperature and thus fail to take preventive measures, such as dressing appropriately or using air conditioning or fans
   3. Heat waves can have severe effects in older adults

C. Nursing implications
   1. Keep in mind that nursing goals are to reduce body temperature, to help determine the cause of hyperthermia, and to provide supportive care during hyperthermic episodes
   2. For the patient with mild hyperthermia, nursing interventions include:
      a. Administering cool drinks
      b. Reducing clothing to a minimum
      c. Reducing the patient's activity level
      d. Sponging the patient's face and hands with tepid water
      e. Reducing ambient temperature
   3. For the patient with more severe hyperthermia (body temperature above 103° F [39.4° C]), nursing interventions include:
      a. Undressing the patient and covering with sheets or towels moistened with ice chips and water
      b. Applying ice packs to the patient's head and back of the neck
      c. Sponging the patient with tepid water, then directing dry air over the patient to promote cooling

4. Measure the patient's rectal temperature frequently during all cooling measures to prevent too rapid a temperature change, which may affect blood pressure and pulse
5. If the patient starts to shiver, stop the cooling process immediately; shivering will raise body temperature to the previous level
6. Suspect infection in a hyperthermic patient if ambient temperature is below 80° F (26.6° C); observe for signs and symptoms of urinary tract infection and respiratory infection
7. Listen and comfort the patient who experienced hallucinations or delusions during hyperthermia
8. Help prevent hyperthermia by taking measures to prevent infection, promoting hydration, and teaching older adults how to protect themselves during high ambient temperatures
9. Advise older adults to avoid direct sunlight, wear lightweight clothing, use fans, drink cool beverages, eat light foods, get adequate rest, and avoid physical exertion when the ambient temperature is high

IV. Altitude illness

A. General information
1. High altitudes may cause hypotensive changes in older adults who are not acclimated to these conditions
2. Older adults living at high altitudes are less likely to experience altitude-related illnesses because they have become acclimated to the altitude
3. High-altitude pulmonary edema causes such signs and symptoms as increasingly severe dyspnea, tachycardia, persistent cough, noisy gurgling respirations, weakness, orthopnea, hemoptysis, rhonchi, and crackles
4. High-altitude cerebral edema, another serious altitude-related illness, causes such signs and symptoms as increasingly severe headaches, confusion, emotional lability, hallucinations, ataxia, and weakness

B. Contributing factors
1. Older adults with cardiac or respiratory problems may be unable to tolerate a high altitude even if they are acclimated to it
2. Strenuous physical exercise at high altitudes may cause unusual or unfamiliar symptoms in anyone, particularly older adults

C. Nursing implications
1. Keep in mind that the goal of nursing care is to prevent altitude illness
2. Advise older adults with cardiac and respiratory problems to take special precautions when traveling at high altitudes
3. Be aware that interventions for a patient with altitude illness include administering supplemental oxygen, as ordered, and removing the patient to a lower elevation

4. Caution older adults living at high altitudes to avoid strenuous physical exercise

V. Fires and burns

A. General information
    1. Burns may cause severe disability in older adults because healing slows with age
    2. Smoke inhalation is particularly dangerous in older adults with respiratory disorders or decreased vital capacity
    3. In institutional settings with a high risk of accidental fire, staff and residents should conduct advance planning and ongoing training on fire emergency procedures
    4. Fear of fire and of being trapped in a fire because of mobility problems are serious concerns for older adults

B. Contributing factors
    1. Decreased sense of smell impairs the older adult's ability to detect smoke and gas
    2. Older adults may overload old circuitry in their homes or lack the visual acuity to detect frayed electrical cords on lamps and appliances
    3. Decreased sensitivity to heat and pain predisposes older adults to accidental burns
    4. Smoking in bed, a common cause of fires, is particularly hazardous for the older adult

C. Nursing implications
    1. Keep in mind that the nursing goal is to prevent fires and burns
    2. Encourage older adults to use smoke detectors and to check smoke detector batteries regularly
    3. Warn older adults of the hazards posed by extra heating devices, kerosene stoves, gas and electric heaters, and exposed steam pipes
    4. Instruct older adults not to wear loose-fitting clothing when cooking because it may catch on fire
    5. Advise older adults to make sure heating pads, hot water bottles, and electric blankets are well covered to prevent burns; urge them to use these devices with extreme caution
    6. Teach older adults to adjust water heater thermostats so that water from the faucet will not scald them

VI. Medication use

A. General information
    1. Older adults are more susceptible to drug-induced illness and adverse drug effects than younger adults
    2. Sedatives, hypoglycemic agents, cardiac drugs, and diuretics are the drugs most commonly prescribed for older adults

AGE-RELATED CHANGES AFFECTING DRUG ACTION

This table lists age-related changes in pharmacokinetics and drug activity along with their corresponding effects.

PROCESS	AGE-RELATED CHANGE	EFFECT
Drug absorption	Decrease in gastric acid	Decrease in drug solubility
	Reduction in mesenteric blood flow	Possible reduction in drug absorption
	Reduction in size of absorbing surface	Possible reduction in drug absorption
	Impairment in enzyme systems responsible for intestinal epithelial membrane transport	Possible reduction in drug absorption
Drug distribution	Reduction in total body water and lean body mass per kilogram of body weight; increase in body fat	Increased distribution of drugs with high lipid solubility; decreased distribution of drugs with high water solubility
	Reduction in serum albumin	Reduced amount of available protein for highly protein-bound drugs
	Blood flow changes	Changes in drug distribution
	Changes in tissue permeability and thickness	Changes in drug distribution and elimination
Drug metabolism	Diminished kidney function, especially glomerular filtration rates and blood flow	Increased risk of drug accumulation and toxicity; prolonged drug half-life
	Diminished liver function	Increased drug toxicity; prolonged drug half-life
Drug activity	Altered receptor sites and related tissue responses	Changes in intensity of drug action (increased or decreased)

Used with permission from Stolley, J., Buckwalter, K., and Fjordbak, B., "Introgenesis in the Elderly," *Journal of Gerontological Nursing* 17(9): 13, 1991.

3. The four processes of pharmacokinetics — DRUG ABSORPTION, DRUG DISTRIBUTION, DRUG METABOLISM, and DRUG EXCRETION — are altered in older adults (see *Age-related changes affecting drug action*)
   a. Absorption of drugs administered by the oral, intramuscular (I.M.), and subcutaneous routes is altered in older adults

(1) Impaired absorption of oral drugs may stem from mucosal atrophy, decreased gastric emptying, reduced splanchnic blood flow, duodenal diverticula, and decreased gastrointestinal (GI) motility

(2) Decreased gastric acid secretion and higher pH may affect ionization and absorption of some oral drugs

(3) Absorption of I.M. and subcutaneous drugs may be delayed from reduced blood flow and altered capillary wall permeability

b. Alterations in drug distribution result from various age-related changes

(1) Decreases in body weight and total body water lead to higher plasma concentrations of water-soluble drugs

(2) A decrease in lean body mass and an increase in body fat causes increased concentration of lipid-soluble drugs, which accumulate in fat and prolong drug action

(3) A decrease in circulating plasma albumin reduces the number of protein-binding sites for drugs

(a) Consequently, levels of unbound pharmacologically active drugs increase

(b) This heightens the risk of adverse reactions and drug toxicity

c. Alterations in drug metabolism increase the risk of drug accumulation and toxicity and may prolong half-life

d. Alterations in drug excretion also result from age-related changes

(1) Most drugs are eliminated or excreted through the kidneys; because renal function declines with age, drug excretion becomes slower and less efficient

(2) Common medical conditions in older adults, such as dehydration, congestive heart failure, pneumonia, urinary tract infection, and renal disease, further impair drug excretion

4. Drugs frequently misused by older adults include sleeping pills, antianxiety agents, pain medications, and laxatives

B. Related considerations

1. The incidence of drug interactions increases with age and the number of drugs prescribed

2. Response to drug therapy is determined by individual variables, such as drug history; body mass; and physiologic and psychological status

3. Older adults commonly have multiple pathologic conditions that necessitate use of multiple medications; POLYPHARMACY increases the risk of adverse drug reactions

a. Older adults may obtain prescriptions from different physicians

b. They may use over-the-counter (OTC) drugs without informing the physician

c. They may share drugs with neighbors, relatives, and friends

4. Acute and chronic illnesses may alter pharmacokinetics further in older adults
5. Drug omission is common among older adults because of complicated drug therapy schedules, memory deficits, insufficient income to purchase drugs, unpleasant side effects, and fear that drugs may be habit-forming
6. Adverse reactions to drugs, such as confusion, forgetfulness, weakness, and anorexia, may be mistaken for normal age-related changes

C. Nursing implications
1. Keep in mind that the nursing goal is to assist the patient with responsible medication use
2. Obtain a complete medical history, including use of OTC drugs
3. Verify the patient's ability to read
4. Monitor the patient's response to drugs and observe for adverse reactions
5. Monitor plasma concentrations of such drugs as digoxin, antiarrhythmics, antidepressants, and theophylline to prevent toxicity
6. Act as an advocate for physician review of patient prescriptions every 6 months; instruct the patient to take a list of all current medications to physician visits
7. Determine if the patient is taking any medications incorrectly by finding out which medications the patient takes and how the patient takes them (for instance, taking OTC laxatives with prescribed medications at bedtime may be inappropriate because of increased bowel transit time)
8. Encourage the patient to use the same pharmacy for all prescriptions to prevent duplication of medications
9. Recognize patients at high risk for adverse reactions, such as those who see several physicians; those who live alone; and those with multiple chronic illnesses, renal failure, frail health, small build, female sex, history of adverse reactions or drug allergies, altered mental status, or financial problems
10. Ensure that the patient and family know how to use drugs properly
    a. Teach the patient to take all drugs in the prescribed manner; for instance, instruct the patient not to crush or mix drugs with fruit juice unless appropriate
    b. Instruct the patient to place capsules on the front of the tongue and tablets on the back of the tongue for easier swallowing
    c. Instruct the patient to maintain a list of all medications
    d. Teach the patient how to recognize side effects of all prescribed drugs and to report any side effect
    e. Teach the patient to recognize drug limitations
    f. Help the patient set realistic expectations for drug therapy
11. Use appropriate patient teaching techniques
    a. Recognize and address language barriers

   b. Use cognitive, psychomotor, and affective learning objectives
   c. Provide both oral and written instructions (for instance, tape pills to a card to provide a visual aid)
   d. Specify the name and purpose of each drug, administration method and times, proper storage, foods and activities to avoid or use, how long to use each medication, information on adverse reactions and procedures to follow if adverse reactions occur, and refill procedures
   e. Provide follow-up teaching
   f. Establish a predischarge training program for managing drug schedules
   g. Provide patient teaching individually or in small groups
   h. Design materials that help counteract any sensory impairments or memory deficits
   i. Use audiovisual aids
   j. Adjust drug administration instructions to the patient's life-style and habits
12. Inform the patient about assistive devices or special provisions, if necessary, and encourage the patient to use them
   a. Suggest that the patient request large-print labels on drug containers for easier reading
   b. Recommend that the patient use calendars, check-off systems, or commercial devices (such as Mediset) as reminders to take medications on schedule
   c. Inform the patient that screw-cap or flip-top containers are easier to open than childproof containers
   d. Inform the patient that drugs in liquid form may be easier to swallow

VII. Exercise

A. General information
   1. With age, the ability to exercise and perform physical work declines
   2. Cardiac output also decreases with age, leading to reduced maximum work capacity
   3. An age-related decline in vital capacity limits air movement during exercise, causing the respiratory rate to increase
   4. An individually prescribed and supervised exercise program has multiple benefits for older adults
      a. Improved self-esteem
      b. Increased maximal oxygen uptake, a slower heart rate, and reduced systolic blood pressure
      c. Lower serum catecholamine levels
      d. Reduced adipose tissue and an increased percentage of lean body mass

       e. Increased ratio of high-density lipoproteins to low-density lipoproteins

       f. Improved digestion

       g. Less frequent constipation

       h. Muscle strengthening and toning

       i. Increased cardiovascular function

       j. Increased pulmonary function

       k. Increased interaction and socialization with others

       l. Greater ability to cope with stress

   5. Lack of physical activity may contribute to poor appetite, constipation, fatigue, insomnia, stress, and depression

B. Related considerations

   1. Disease and pain may limit physical activity in older adults

   2. Depression and social isolation may contribute to a decreased activity level in older adults

   3. Older adults with temporary or permanent mobility limitations (such as from stroke, fracture, arthritis, general weakness, and acute or chronic illness) need guidance and encouragement to engage in physical activity

   4. Medication use may influence an older adult's ability to engage in exercise and the physiologic response to exercise

   5. Other factors that affect exercise in older adults include proximity to recreational facilities, income, and customary recreational activities

C. Nursing implications

   1. Keep in mind that the nursing goal is to encourage and assist the patient with an exercise program to strengthen muscle tone, improve flexibility and range of motion, relieve boredom, and reduce social isolation

   2. Advise the patient to obtain physician's approval before starting an exercise program

   3. Keep in mind any special physical conditions and limitations when designing the patient's exercise program

   4. Instruct the patient to begin an exercise program gradually

   5. Monitor the patient carefully during the exercise program

   6. Teach the patient to stay alert for such changes as shortness of breath, abnormal facial coloring, labored breathing, lightheadedness, dizziness, or pain while exercising; instruct the patient to stop exercising if any of these occur

   7. Advise the patient to avoid isometric (static) exercises because these stimulate the vagovagal response and raise blood pressure

VIII. Sleep problems

A. General information

1. Deep sleep (Stages 3 and 4 sleep) and rapid eye movement (REM) sleep decrease with aging
2. Stage 4 sleep plays an essential role in restoring physiologic well-being; REM sleep helps relieve tension and anxiety
3. The significance of decreased Stage 4 sleep in older adults has not been established
4. Older adults normally experience frequent arousals, which may cause a false impression of sleeplessness
5. Frequent arousals and reduced duration of deep sleep alter sleep patterns; however, the older adult's need for sleep does not decrease
6. Lack of sleep leads to fatigue, irritability, and increased sensitivity to pain
7. Napping typically increases with age; it provides rest, relaxation, and compensation for loss of sleep at night
8. The incidence of SLEEP APNEA increases with age and is associated with cardiac arrhythmias and sudden death in older adults
9. Hypnotic drugs reduce REM sleep

B. Contributing factors

1. Depression is the most common cause of sleep disturbance in older adults
2. Minimal environmental stimulation, a change in daily routine, boredom, or extended napping during the day may contribute to insomnia
3. Persistent physical symptoms, such as leg cramps, pain, coughing, and frequent urination, also may contribute to insomnia
4. Other factors that may affect sleep include nightmares, worry, and bereavement

C. Nursing implications

1. Keep in mind that the nursing goal is to promote restful sleep
2. Assess and evaluate the patient's sleep history
   a. Current and past sleep patterns
   b. Changes in sleep patterns
   c. Napping patterns
   d. Exercise and activity level
   e. Diet and use of alcohol, drugs, and caffeine
3. Teach the patient about age-related changes in sleep patterns
4. Advise the patient to maintain a quiet, restful environment conducive to sleep and to follow usual bedtime rituals
5. Encourage the patient to exercise early in the day to prevent overstimulation at bedtime

6. For a hospitalized patient, promote comfort by ensuring proper positioning; administering pain medication; providing sufficient warmth; maintaining the patient's usual bedtime rituals to the extent possible; and promoting relaxation by giving back rubs or foot rubs and offering warm milk or a glass of wine, if possible

IX. Leisure activities

A. General information
1. Adequate preparation for retirement may promote adjustment to increased leisure time
2. General health status and attitudes and feelings about retirement help predict an older adult's satisfaction with retirement
3. Typically, four phases of adjustment follow retirement
   a. Phase 1: retirement event, luncheon, or party followed by exhilaration, then a letdown
   b. Phase 2 ("honeymoon" phase): experimentation with new activities to help forge a new life-style
   c. Phase 3: disenchantment with retirement
   d. Phase 4: emergence of new patterns that develop into a satisfying routine
4. Leisure activities should be self-determined and pleasurable and should contribute to a sense of self-worth
5. Choice of leisure activities is influenced by:
   a. Age
   b. Health
   c. Social network
   d. Income
   e. Location
   f. Work role
   g. Family structure
   h. Changes in health, energy level, and sensory function
   i. Personal preference

B. Related considerations
1. Older adults tend to maintain the same patterns of leisure activity that they established early in life
2. Some older adults may view retirement as a crisis, with loss of the self-esteem previously derived from work success
3. Older adults who have lived a highly structured life-style may experience anxiety from the increase in unstructured time
4. Retirement may cause a decrease in income, possibly limiting one's choice of activities

C. Nursing implications
1. Keep in mind that the nursing goal is to help the patient adjust to increased leisure time

2. Encourage older adults to plan for retirement adequately in advance, including anticipated leisure activities
3. Advise the patient to plan some regular activity outside the home to maintain social interaction and self-esteem
4. Assist the patient who prefers a structured life-style to develop new daily routines
5. Refer the patient to local senior citizen centers and community recreational facilities, if appropriate
6. Keep in mind that day-care programs may be available for older adults with physical or mental impairments
7. Inform the patient about senior citizen groups and organizations that arrange trips and offer discounts; these may hold particular interest for older adults who enjoy traveling and socializing

X. Sexual function

A. General information
1. Sexuality is an important aspect to consider when caring for older adults
2. Sexuality includes such behaviors as touching, kissing, handholding, and massages
3. Sexual interest, activity, and needs persist well into old age, provided the older adult remains in good health and has an interested and interesting partner
4. Regular stimulation through intercourse or masturbation helps maintain interest in sex
5. Sexual problems in older adults commonly result from emotional or social factors rather than biological or organic conditions
6. Sexual function in older adults is affected by age-related changes in erection and ejaculation in men and by vaginal lubrication in women
7. Older adults may take longer to achieve arousal
8. Intimacy, companionship, and physical closeness are especially important to older adults

B. Related considerations
1. Past sexual activity and enjoyment are the best predictors of sexual behavior in older adults
2. Barriers to sexual expression may involve health status, cultural attitudes, opportunity, and the patient's sexual history
3. An older adult may cease sexual activity because of a partner's illness or death, disinterest, monotony, or substitution of a satisfying nonsexual activity
4. Fear of failure during sexual intercourse may cause an older adult to avoid sexual activity
5. Lack of privacy is a common obstacle to sexual expression among older adults, especially those who live with adult children or in institutions

6. A history of heart disease — especially myocardial infarction — may cause an older adult to avoid sex from fear of another acute episode
7. Arthritis may be painful enough to limit sexual activity
8. Illness and medications may reduce libido and cause erectile problems in older men; diabetes mellitus may cause impotence
9. Prostatectomy usually does not impair sexual capacity or enjoyment
10. Common gynecologic problems that may limit sexual activity in older women include senile vaginitis, vulvitis, perineal pruritus, uterine prolapse, cystocele, and rectocele

C. Nursing implications
1. Keep in mind that nursing goals are to provide information about sexuality and to assist older adults in being comfortable about sexual function
2. Help older adults become aware of their beliefs and attitudes toward sexuality and aging
3. Teach older adults about age-related changes in sexual function
4. Assist older adults with resolving sexual issues
5. Incorporate the patient's sexual history into the nursing assessment
6. Protect and maintain the sexual rights of older adults
7. Refer the patient with sexual problems for a medical work-up and counseling
8. Advise the patient with a history of heart disease to avoid sexual relations after a large meal, during extreme environmental temperatures, in anxiety-provoking situations, and when feelings of anger or resentment exist
9. Recommend position changes during sexual intercourse to alleviate joint pain
10. As appropriate, recommend variations in positions used for sexual intercourse (such as more passive positions for a patient with a history of a coronary condition or cerebrovascular accident)
11. Teach the patient about the effects of drugs and alcohol on sexual function (such as decreased libido and difficulty in maintaining an erection)

XI. Dental health and oral hygiene

A. General information
1. Tooth loss may result from tooth decay (dental caries) or periodontal disease; it is not a normal effect of aging
2. Periodontal disease, a common problem among older adults, causes inflammation leading to degeneration of tissues supporting the teeth; signs and symptoms include:
   a. Pain
   b. Swelling
   c. Loose teeth
   d. Fetid breath

　　　e. A bad taste
　3. Wearing away of teeth over a lifetime may result from cumulative
　　　factors, such as:
　　　a. Attrition (grinding from tooth-to-tooth contact, as in chewing)
　　　b. Abrasion (rubbing away by friction, as from a toothbrush)
　　　c. Erosion (loss of tooth enamel resulting from a chemical process,
　　　　such as emesis, not from bacteria)
　4. Approximately 50% of adults over age 65 are edentulous (lacking some
　　　or all natural teeth)
　5. About 90% of oral cancer cases occur after age 45; the typical victim
　　　is a man who is a heavy smoker or who chews tobacco
　6. LEUKOPLAKIA, a precancerous condition, may develop from chronic
　　　mouth irritation

B. Related considerations
　1. Decreased saliva production and use of drugs that cause dry mouth
　　　make older adults vulnerable to tooth decay and dryness and cracking
　　　of the oral mucosa
　2. Age-related changes of the oral mucosa (such as epithelial thinning
　　　and drying) predispose older adults to mucosal injury
　3. Breathing through the mouth contributes to dryness of the oral
　　　mucosa and increases the risk of tissue irritation and damage
　4. Certain drugs may induce changes in the oral mucosa
　5. Decreased sensitivity to warm liquids or foods may cause mouth
　　　burns and other oral lesions
　6. Dentures may cause such problems as sore mouth, improper fit,
　　　difficulty chewing, and inflammatory hyperplasia (tissue flaps around
　　　denture edges)
　7. Older adults may not obtain regular dental care because of anxiety,
　　　unaffordable cost, transportation problems, and lack of a perceived
　　　need
　8. Routine nursing care may neglect oral hygiene

C. Nursing implications
　1. Keep in mind that the nursing goal is to prevent tooth loss and
　　　periodontal disease by promoting self-care and, if needed, assistance
　　　with oral hygiene
　2. Be sure to include oral hygiene as part of routine nursing care
　3. If the patient cannot perform routine mouth care, clean the mouth
　　　with a soft-bristle toothbrush and dental floss to remove plaque
　4. If the patient cannot tolerate brushing or flossing, moisten and clean
　　　the mouth with normal saline solution; avoid solutions containing
　　　alcohol
　5. To remove viscous secretions or dried mucus, use sodium bicarbonate
　　　(10 ml in 100 ml of normal saline solution) or hydrogen peroxide
　　　solutions ($1/4$ to $1/2$ H_2O_2); be sure to remove these solutions from the
　　　mouth with water or saline solution

6. Teach the patient proper brushing and flossing techniques
7. Instruct the patient about proper denture care and oral hygiene
8. Encourage the patient to obtain preventive dental care through regular check-ups every 6 to 12 months
9. Advise the patient to remove dentures at bedtime

XII. Nutrition

A. General information
   1. Many health problems in older adults result from poor nutrition
   2. Nutritional status affects overall health status and energy level
   3. Nutritional deficiencies usually result from inappropriate food selections rather than inadequate food intake
   4. Common dietary deficiencies among older adults include protein, vitamins C and D, folic acid, calcium, and iron deficiencies
   5. Older adults gain weight more easily than younger adults from a decreased basal metabolic rate and reduced physical activity
   6. Although older adults need fewer calories than younger adults, requirements for vitamins, minerals, and protein remain essentially the same

B. Related considerations
   1. Impaired thirst sensation may cause decreased fluid intake in older adults
   2. Financial resources may determine the amount of food an older adult consumes
   3. Immobility may limit an older adult's ability to obtain and prepare food
   4. Immobility and lack of exercise contribute to poor appetite in older adults
   5. Loneliness and depression may impair an older adult's eating habits
   6. Dental problems, such as missing or loose teeth and poorly fitting dentures, affect the ability to chew and the types of foods an older adult eats
   7. A diminished sense of smell and taste may decrease the stimulation to eat
   8. Impaired digestion (from age-related changes in stomach or bowel function) may affect nutritional status
   9. Institutionalized older adults may lose interest in food from a bland or monotonous diet
   10. Complex therapeutic diets may be hard for older adults to understand and prepare, leading to noncompliance
   11. Ethnic and cultural preferences influence food choices

C. Nursing implications
   1. Keep in mind that the nursing goal is to maintain optimal nutritional status through education and diet provisions that incorporate the patient's food preferences and cultural customs
   2. Limit dietary changes to those necessary for health
   3. Teach the patient about proper use of vitamin and mineral supplements
   4. Teach the patient the principles of good nutrition and explain the rationale for any prescribed therapeutic diet
   5. Assist with meal planning, keeping the patient's food preferences and cultural customs in mind
   6. Recognize the personal and social aspects of eating meals
   7. Inform the patient of dietary recommendations that may reduce the risk of cancer and heart disease
      a. Increased consumption of fresh fruits and vegetables and whole grains
      b. Avoidance of foods containing refined and processed sugar
      c. Decreased consumption of processed foods
      d. Reduced consumption of fats
      e. Limited sodium intake
   8. Counsel low-income older adults to contact the local Department of Social Service to find out if they qualify for food stamps
   9. Suggest that the patient who lives alone set an attractive table and prepare an enjoyable meal; mention that a pet, a good book, or a television or radio program may increase meal enjoyment

XIII. Nursing interventions for common problems in hospitalized older adults

A. Poor eating habits
   1. Help the patient fill out menu choices to ensure nutritious selections
   2. If possible, encourage the patient to get out of bed to eat or to be with others at meals
   3. Make sure the patient's dentures are in place during meals
   4. Ask the family to bring in the seasonings the patient uses at home; use salt substitutes, if indicated, to enhance flavor
   5. Provide various flavorings for dietary supplements and formula feedings
   6. Adjust meals to the patient's life-style and daily routines
   7. Be aware that brightly colored foods add interest and variety to meals and that large portions may overwhelm the patient
   8. Make sure meal trays are served promptly to keep hot foods hot and cold foods cold
   9. Have snacks (such as toast, custard, hot chocolate, and fruit) available at night
   10. Assist with oral hygiene

11. Avoid interrupting meals for tests and medication administration
12. Offer food substitutions when the patient misses a meal
13. Determine if prescribed medications, such as I.V. antibiotics or potassium, are affecting the patient's appetite

B. Urinary incontinence
1. Identify the patient's voiding patterns and offer frequent opportunities for the patient to use the toilet
2. Help the patient use the toilet after meals
3. Maintain the voiding routines that the patient usually follows at home
4. Evaluate the patient's functional abilities (for instance, ability to get up to go to the bathroom)
5. Make sure the patient has access to a bedside commode, if necessary
6. After an incontinence episode, determine if the patient had any forewarning of the need to urinate
7. Know that a recumbent position enhances the action of diuretics (from an increased glomerular filtration rate); plan timing of medication administration, as appropriate, to promote or prevent this effect
8. Consider limiting the patient's consumption of coffee, tea, and other stimulants that may have a diuretic effect
9. Be aware that limiting fluid intake after 8:00 P.M. may help prevent nighttime incontinence
10. Keep in mind that the patient may need to void several times during the night (or more frequently if receiving I.V. therapy)
11. If the patient uses a bedpan, consider keeping it in the bed for quick access
12. Keep a bell or call light within the patient's reach
13. Be aware that urinary catheterization is used only as a last resort for urinary incontinence

C. Fecal incontinence
1. Check for fecal impaction
2. Evaluate the patient's functional ability (for example, ability to get up and walk to the bathroom)
3. Check the patient's medications (antibiotics, for instance, may cause diarrhea)
4. Check the patient's diagnosis; fecal incontinence may result from such pathologic conditions as spinal cancer, stroke, or GI bleeding
5. Check for laxative abuse; keep in mind that patients may ask family members to supply laxatives
6. Determine if the patient is dependent on enemas
7. Institute bowel retraining, if appropriate
8. Consider increasing the bulk and fiber content of the patient's diet

D. Constipation
1. Check the patient's medications for agents that may cause constipation (for example, narcotics)

    2. Monitor fluid intake and increase it, if necessary
    3. Suggest that the patient drink hot water with lemon and honey
    4. Incorporate a regular exercise program into the patient's routine, if possible
    5. Reestablish previous bowel elimination routines (for instance, bowel movements first thing in the morning or after meals)
    6. Keep water available and within the patient's reach
    7. Give extra fluids with medications
    8. Give juices and other fluids between meals
    9. Have the patient use a bedside commode instead of a bedpan when possible
   10. Provide uninterrupted privacy when the patient is trying to have a bowel movement

E. Insomnia
    1. Be aware that hospitalization disrupts sleeping patterns
    2. Provide a night-light and keep the patient's door closed
    3. Make sure the patient is warm enough at night
    4. Decrease noise and other distractions
    5. Make sure the patient uses the toilet before going to bed
    6. Offer a snack
    7. Sit and listen to the patient's concerns
    8. Evaluate whether a change of roommate would be appropriate
    9. Find out what sleep-inducing measures the patient uses at home (for example, reading, listening to music, or drinking hot milk)
   10. Provide a warm washcloth for the patient's hands and face
   11. Offer a backrub
   12. Assess the patient's need for pain medication
   13. Make sure prescribed medications are administered before the patient settles down for the night, if possible
   14. Offer additional pillows or help the patient to a more comfortable bed position
   15. Check to see if the patient's medications contain caffeine
   16. Adjust the patient's sheets, if necessary, making sure that the bottom sheet is smooth
   17. Be aware that the patient may want familiar objects nearby, such as pictures or a clock
   18. Encourage diversionary activities, such as reading or watching television
   19. Help the patient accept the fact that sleep problems may occur from time to time

F. Confusion
    1. Orient the patient to the environment and the equipment in the room to reduce confusion
    2. Use a night-light if the patient seems more confused at night

3. Ask a family member to stay or arrange for someone to sit with the patient, if necessary
4. Recognize that a confused patient may exhibit unusual or inappropriate behavior, such as identifying the nurse as a daughter
5. Be aware that words spoken by a confused patient might have meaning to the patient; however, always try to reorient the patient
6. Find out if the patient needs to use the toilet
7. Place familiar objects where the patient can see them
8. Eliminate or modify pain and sleep medications, if possible
9. Ask the patient's family what techniques they use to cope with confusion at home; try to adapt successful techniques to the hospital environment
10. Stay calm; staff anxiety may increase the patient's anxiety
11. Encourage the patient to reminisce because this helps reduce confusion and resulting anxiety
12. Reduce environmental stimuli

G. Pain
1. Determine what type of pain the patient is experiencing (for instance, chest pain or gas pain)
2. Implement appropriate interventions after identifying the cause of pain
3. Keep in mind that multiple causes of pain may exist but that the most frequent cause is musculoskeletal
4. Use warm towels and massage
5. Use a trapeze to facilitate movement
6. Have the patient contract and relax each muscle group
7. Adjust the bed position and pillows
8. Check for factors contributing to pain, such as constipation or leg cramps
9. If possible, use nursing interventions to reduce pain (such as relaxation exercises) before giving sleep medications
10. Identify psychological concerns that may make pain or discomfort worse at night; be aware that such interventions as listening, stroking, and providing companionship or diversionary activities may help
11. Get the patient interested in something, such as television, games, puzzles, reading, or reminiscing

Points to remember

Falls, fire and burns, hypothermia, and hyperthermia are major safety problems for older adults.

Medication misuse is a common problem among older adults.

Exercise helps counteract some problems experienced by older adults, such as immobility.

Sleep patterns change with age.

Medications may contribute to sleep disturbances.

Older adults may need counseling to broaden opportunities for leisure activities.

Sexual interest and activity normally continue into older adulthood.

Nutritional problems among older adults may result directly from dental problems.

Glossary

The following terms are defined in Appendix A, page 194.

drug absorption	leukoplakia
drug distribution	polypharmacy
drug excretion	sleep apnea
drug metabolism	

Study questions

To evaluate your understanding of this chapter, answer the following questions in the space provided; then compare your responses with the correct answers in Appendix B, pages 204 and 205.

1. What are two physical factors contributing to falls in older adults? _____

   _____

   _____

2. The nurse should use which method to monitor temperature in an older adult with hypothermia? _____

   _____

3. How does heat exhaustion differ from heat stroke? _____

   _____

4. The nurse should expect which assessment findings in an older adult with high-altitude cerebral edema? _____

   _____

5. What are two factors that predispose an older adult to fires and burns?

   _____

   _____

6. Which pharmacokinetic processes are altered in older adults? _____

   _____

   _____

7. The nurse should advise older adults to avoid which type of exercise?

   _____

   _____

8. What is the most common cause of sleep disturbance in older adults?

   _____

   _____

Study questions *(continued)*

9. What occurs during each of the four phases of adjustment to retirement?

_____

_____

10. What are the best predictors of sexual behavior in older adults? _____

_____

_____

11. How should the nurse perform oral care for the patient who cannot tolerate brushing or flossing the teeth? _____

_____

12. What is a common cause of nutritional deficiencies in older adults?

_____

_____

13. What are three common problems in hospitalized older adults? _____

_____

_____

CHAPTER 8

Resources for Support

Learning objectives

Check off the following items once you've mastered them:

☐ Identify the role that adult children play in caring for elderly parents.

☐ Describe two community-based services designed to meet the nutritional, housing, or transportation needs of older adults.

☐ Identify the major differences between skilled nursing facilities and intermediate-care facilities.

☐ Name two reasons for the growing interest in home health care.

I. Family support

A. General information

1. Health status affects an older adult's relationships, social contacts, self-care activities, and living arrangements
2. Illness and hospitalization decrease the older adult's functional capacity
3. Loss of functional capacity makes the older adult more dependent and increases the need for family involvement in care
4. Although most older adults are independent, approximately 33% require help
5. The family unit is the basic social unit and the primary support system for older adults; besides providing care for older adults, families provide affection and social interaction
6. The role of family members changes as an older adult ages
7. Older adults prefer to live near their children but not with them
   a. Roughly 84% of older adults live less than 1 hour away from a family member
   b. About 18% of older adults live with one of their children
8. Most elderly couples live alone, with the spouse serving as primary caregiver
   a. Children assist with care of an elderly parent
   b. After the caregiving spouse dies, children become the primary caregivers
      (1) Children typically provide care to avoid institutionalization of an elderly parent
      (2) In many cases, the functionally impaired parent is maintained at home
9. Other relatives and friends typically do not have the caregiving duties and responsibilities of immediate family members; however, they may act as informed peripheral caregivers
10. Approximately 80% of the care of old-old adults is provided by family members
11. About 40% of persons age 50 to 60 have a surviving parent; about 20% of persons age 60 to 70 have a surviving parent
12. Demographic studies show that fewer children are available to share the care of an elderly parent despite the increasing number of four-generation families
13. About 50% of women aged 45 to 64 work and serve as primary caregivers to an older adult (in addition to their other roles)
14. Caregiving places added physical and mental stress on the family of the older adult
    a. Physical care places the greatest demand on family members
    b. Caregiver stress results from multiple demands, isolation, loneliness, and low morale

    c. A caregiving spouse is vulnerable to health problems from energy drain

    d. Adult children caring for elderly parents have their own health problems, developmental activities, and losses to deal with

    e. Some family members cannot and should not be caregivers

    f. Unresolved relationship problems within a family contribute to strain and magnify the crisis

    g. Family members may express guilt and anger; also, they may be distressed by the nature of the older adult's health problems

B. Nursing implications

  1. Assess the ability of family members to act as caregivers

  2. Prepare adult children for a shift to dependency by their aging parents

  3. Recognize the interrelationships, independence, and reciprocity of family members' roles

  4. Support the older adult's efforts to participate in self-care and decision making

  5. Establish a relationship with the patient's family and support all family members

  6. Involve family members in the care of an older adult who is hospitalized or institutionalized, if they desire

  7. Help the family to identify and use available resources, such as RESPITE CARE and counseling

  8. Teach family members about the aging process and potential physical and mental problems of elderly parents

  9. Help family members negotiate sharing of care activities

II. Community-based resources

A. Nutrition

  1. Food programs are designed to improve or maintain nutrition and to maintain older adults' independence

  2. Such programs also provide social contact and an opportunity for older adults to develop relationships with others

  3. Eligibility for food programs may be based on ability or inability to pay

  4. Quality of service may determine an older adult's participation in a food program

  5. Federally funded nutrition sites provide one CONGREGATE MEAL per day

  6. Meals on Wheels delivers meals to homebound persons

  7. Religious organizations and community groups may provide meals to older adults

  8. Food stamp programs are available to some older adults

  9. Loneliness, not lack of money, may pose a major nutritional problem for older adults who have trouble eating properly when alone

B. Housing
1. Inadequate income is the major factor contributing to housing problems among older adults
2. About 70% of older adults live in single homes; about 30% live in hotels, rental units, public housing, and institutions
3. Many older adults need money to modify their home so that they can remain there
4. When an older adult no longer can live at home for economic or health reasons, alternative housing choices include age-segregated or age-integrated housing complexes, public housing for older adults, shared housing, and congregate housing
   a. The trend is toward housing alternatives that provide continuity of care, such as life-care facilities
   b. In rural areas, few alternatives exist and housing conditions are poorest
5. Day-care and social programs at community centers that provide daytime care or supervision may avert a housing crisis by enabling an older adult to remain at home or with family members instead of relocating to an institution
6. Older adults remaining at home should be made aware that 24-hour emergency medical response services, such as LifeCall, are available
7. Less support exists for housing than for other needs, such as provision of meals, cleaning, transportation, and medication-giving

C. Transportation
1. About 8.3 million older adults drive cars; accidents involving such drivers are twice as likely to be fatal as those involving younger drivers
2. Many older adults depend on friends and relatives for transportation
3. Transportation problems of older adults include lack of a vehicle, inability to drive, insufficient money to keep a car, and distance from health care providers and other services
4. Alternatives to driving include reduced-fare taxis, public transportation programs, volunteer drivers, dial-a-ride programs, and chartered bus excursions
   a. Volunteers who transport older adults may have problems obtaining insurance coverage
   b. Public policy considerations include the need for more reduced fares and barrier-free transportation
5. Lack of transportation may lead to social withdrawal, poor nutrition, lack of medical care, and loss of independence
6. Minority and rural older adults have more transportation problems than others
7. Programs to supplement transportation do not address transportation for pleasure

D. Education
  1. Education builds self-esteem, decreases isolation, and maintains intellectual involvement in older adults
  2. Older adults may take or teach classes
     a. They may qualify for reduced or waived tuition
     b. Relevancy of class topics is important to older adults
     c. Subjects of interest to many older adults include health, budget and insurance information, arts, and new skills (such as crafts or home repair)
     d. High schools, colleges, and universities may offer special programs for older adults; such programs may be for credit or noncredit and may be short or full-course offerings
     e. Elderhostels offer noncredit courses on a live-in basis on residential campuses
     f. Older adults usually prefer discovery learning (exploring a topic at one's own pace) because it reduces anxiety
  3. Factors that may limit an older adult's participation in education include cost, location, transportation, and safety
  4. Older adults who decide to pursue a degree may need help with study skills
  5. Illiteracy may prevent some older adults from taking classes
  6. Older adults can obtain videotapes, audio cassettes, and large-print books from libraries

E. Nursing implications for all community-based resources
  1. Carefully assess the patient's needs (such as nutrition, transportation, housing, and education)
  2. Be aware of available resources and refer patients appropriately
  3. Act as an advocate to maintain and initiate programs and needs assessment for program development
  4. Help the patient resolve cost, safety, and support issues that may interfere with participation
  5. Keep in mind that community-based programs may meet an older adult's needs and thus help prevent institutionalization

III. Acute care resources

A. General information
  1. Acute care usually is provided in hospitals
     a. The patient must need full-day nursing care to be admitted to a hospital
     b. The hospital environment causes stress that affects the patient's adaptation
     c. The hospital environment presents cure-versus-care issues for the nurse
     d. Length of stay is an economic issue because of the prospective payment system of diagnostic-related groups (DRGs)

2. Short-term, less intensive acute care may be provided in the physician's office rather than a hospital

B. Related considerations
   1. The focus of acute care is on curing and healing
   2. Both complex health problems and normal age-related changes necessitate adjustments in care of older adults

IV. Long-term care resources

A. General information
   1. Long-term care (LTC) is aimed at meeting the increasing dependency and support needs of older adults with chronic physical or mental conditions
   2. The goal of LTC is to promote an optimal level of physical, psychological, and social functioning
   3. LTC services include diagnostic, preventive, therapeutic, rehabilitative, supportive, and maintenance services
      a. LTC services are provided in various settings, both institutional and noninstitutional
      b. Use of LTC services is based on medical need, functional status, availability of family and financial support, and the patient's living arrangements
      c. The decision about which LTC services to use is based on acceptability, availability, and affordability
      d. Availability of LTC resources is the major determinant of use
   4. LTC facilities may be public (government run), voluntary (nonprofit), or proprietary (for profit)
   5. Major problems associated with LTC include fragmented resources, gaps in services, multiple funding sources, and limited community-based alternatives to institutional care
   6. Limited reimbursement for care also is a major concern (for more information on this topic, see Chapter 10)
      a. LTC insurance is becoming available
      b. Medicare and Medicaid reimburse for LTC only under certain conditions
      c. To a large extent, personal financial resources must be used to pay for LTC
   7. Quality of care is a major issue
      a. Few registered nurses work in LTC settings
      b. Staff members receive little education on aging
      c. Each state sets its own staff requirements
   8. Medicare and Medicaid officials survey LTC facilities
   9. No national LTC policy exists; definitions of types of LTC facilities and programs vary from state to state

10. Key differences between LTCs and hospitals include length of stay, type of care, perception of the quality of care, and prestige accorded to the staff by society

B. Types of LTC
 1. LTC SKILLED NURSING FACILITIES (SNFs) are nursing homes that deliver LTC to patients who are chronically ill or disabled and who need full-day nursing care; these facilities provide physical, occupational, and recreational therapy and social services
 2. LTC INTERMEDIATE-CARE FACILITIES are nursing homes that provide custodial care and personal care services to patients requiring less than 24-hour-a-day nursing care
 3. LTC also can be delivered by home health agencies
    a. Home health care provides an alternative to institutional LTC
    b. Over 3,000 home health agencies exist
    c. These agencies may be directed by private agencies or hospitals
    d. Interest in maintaining older adults at home is growing for financial and humanitarian reasons
    e. In rural areas, fewer home health care agencies and services are available
    f. Many home health services are limited by reimbursement problems; this is a national concern
       (1) Medicare and Medicaid strictly limit reimbursable services and do not pay for LTC home services
       (2) Home health care for chronically ill patients is paid for with private resources
 4. Certain other types of facilities also deliver LTC
    a. Such facilities include rest homes, homes for the aged, and convalescent homes
    b. Care provided by these facilities ranges from a PROTECTIVE ENVIRONMENT to personal care and some skilled care
 5. Other alternatives to institutional LTC include day care, respite care, and foster care

C. Nursing implications
 1. Help older adults and their families explore LTC options before the need for LTC arises
 2. Assist with identifying the appropriate level of care for the patient
    a. Assess the patient's health and functional status
    b. Determine the range of services the patient needs
    c. Match resources with the patient's needs; provide the least restrictive environment possible
 3. Support decision making by the patient's family
 4. Help the patient and family select the best LTC facility
    a. Use such criteria as the amount of privacy offered, patient and staff relationships, types of daily activities offered, and staff-to-patient ratios

      b. Consider other selection criteria, including cost; opportunity for family involvement in care plan and activities; Medicare and/or Medicaid certification; current licensure; and Medicare and/or Medicaid survey findings on the facility's safety, environment, comfort, financial status, and medical, rehabilitative, pharmaceutical, dental, and nutritional services

      c. Use the checklist provided by the U.S. Department of Health and Human Services for selection criteria; the local health department may assist with referral to the facility

  5. Plan for the patient's transition to the LTC facility

  6. Assist the patient and family in adjusting to placement in an LTC facility

      a. Be aware that placement causes stress and may represent loss of privacy and control to the patient

      b. Keep in mind that the family may feel guilty

      c. Know that the patient and family may view placement as the last stage before death

  7. Monitor quality of care in the LTC facility using nursing standards and standards of external reviewers, such as Medicare

  8. Review the statement of residents' rights with the patient and family, if the facility has such a document

  9. Act as an advocate for better staff-to-patient ratios in LTC facilities

V. Community health care

A. General information

  1. Community health care provides services in the context of family and community

  2. Community health care involves health promotion, treatment, rehabilitation, service provision, and provision and evaluation of primary care services

  3. Community health care services are provided in such settings as private offices, homes, schools, workplaces, and ambulatory care centers

  4. Community health care services for older adults commonly include rehabilitation services, adult day care, respite care, and home health care

  5. Older adults have specific needs for community health care

      a. Available and accessible home services for acute and chronic care, including highly technical and holistic posthospital care

      b. Medication management

      c. Coordinated services between the hospital and home

      d. Coordinated, comprehensive network of community services to maintain the independence of the older adult and family within the health care system for as long as possible

e. Community-based primary, secondary, and tertiary prevention services

B. Nursing implications
1. Help the patient perform developmental tasks of aging, such as finding adequate living quarters (at home, in a retirement community, or with children), adapting to retirement income, securing physical and emotional health protection, and feeling a personal sense of worth
2. Counsel older adults regarding life changes associated with aging
3. Teach older adults about chronic disease and health problem risk factors, such as lack of exercise, smoking, excessive drinking, obesity, diets high in fat and cholesterol, environmental toxins, and accidents
4. Provide the patient with information about community resources for physical and emotional well-being
5. Support the patient's sense of self-responsibility for health
6. Encourage participation of older adults and community members on citizens' councils and political action committees as spokespersons for their age-group needs
7. Instruct older adults about medication schedules, therapeutic and adverse drug effects, and safe use of prescribed and over-the-counter medications
8. Counsel older adults on effective and productive uses of time
9. Support the patient's family as they adapt to an aging member
10. Counsel and teach families about the normal aging process as well as specific diseases and health problems
11. Conduct a comprehensive health assessment of the patient's body systems and status within the family and community
12. Conduct community screening programs to detect health problems in older adults
13. Teach the patient about treatments, therapies, and medication
14. Supervise ancillary health care personnel who provide patient services in the home
15. Coordinate nursing services with those provided by other health team members
16. Counsel the patient and family as they adapt to life-style changes brought about by the patient's health problems
17. Help the patient return to the best possible level of function
18. Inform the patient and family of appropriate community resources
19. Promote a family and community network of support for the patient
20. Initiate rehabilitation strategies during acute illness
21. Assist the patient with follow-up services in the home and community
22. Provide consultation services and educational programs for individuals responsible for care of older adults
23. Support legislation and policies that address the concerns of older adults

Points to remember

Typically, the spouse is the primary caregiver for an older adult.

Families take on added responsibilities for elderly relatives to prevent hospitalization or institutionalization.

The older adult's increased dependency on family members causes role reversals.

Community-based programs can provide support to meet the older adult's needs and help prevent or postpone institutionalization.

Long-term care provides continuity of care to meet the increasing dependency and support needs of older adults.

Glossary

The following terms are defined in Appendix A, page 194.

congregate meals

intermediate-care facility

protective environment

respite care

skilled nursing facility

Study questions

To evaluate your understanding of this chapter, answer the following questions in the space provided; then compare your responses with the correct answers in Appendix B, pages 205 and 206.

1. What are some causes of stress among family members caring for an older adult? _____

   _____

2. Lack of transportation may cause which problems among older adults?

   _____

   _____

3. What is the focus of acute care? _____

   _____

4. How do LTC skilled-nursing facilities differ from LTC intermediate-care facilities? _____

   _____

CHAPTER 9

Legal and Ethical Issues

Learning objectives

Check off the following items once you've mastered them:

☐ Identify one physical sign, one behavioral sign, and one psychological sign of abuse in an older adult.

☐ State the four major effects of crime on older adults.

☐ Identify the most restrictive form of protective service.

☐ Name two requirements for valid informed consent.

I. Abuse or neglect

A. General information
1. ABUSE or NEGLECT is any action or situation that places a person in jeopardy
2. Abuse or neglect may relate to health status, health care, personhood, right to self-determination, property, or income
3. Neglect includes failure to maintain a safe environment
4. Types of abuse and neglect include:
    a. Physical abuse or neglect
    b. Psychological or verbal abuse
    c. Violation of rights
    d. Omission
    e. Material or financial abuse
    f. Sexual abuse or assault
5. In descending order, the most likely perpetrator of abuse of an older adult is:
    a. Spouse
    b. Son or daughter, if no spouse exists
    c. Other caregiver
6. No accurate statistics on abuse or neglect are available
7. Abuse and neglect frequently go unreported; the older adult may refuse to file charges
8. Abuse may be a lifelong pattern of the abuser or an acute response to a situation perceived as intolerable

B. Risk group characteristics
1. The typical victim of physical and psychological abuse is a white woman age 66 to 83 who is not severely ill and whose income is below $7,000
2. The typical victim of physical and psychological neglect is a white person age 72 to 89 who lives with relatives, is physically dependent, and has an income below $7,000
3. The typical victim of financial abuse and neglect is a white person age 72 to 89 who lives with nonrelatives, is not severely ill, and has an income below $7,000
4. The most commonly abused person is an elderly woman with chronic physical or mental impairment who is perceived to be aggressive

C. Signs and symptoms of abuse or neglect
1. Physical findings include:
    a. Unexplained bruises, fractures, or other injuries
    b. Poor hygiene or grooming
    c. Malnutrition
    d. Evidence of inappropriate medication administration
2. Behavioral findings include:
    a. Excessive fear

   b. Compliant or dependent behavior
   c. Self-blame
   d. Avoidance of the abuser's touch
   e. Expression of concern that the abuser is taking the person's money or property
   f. Lack of needed supervision
   g. Lack of money, transportation, or other support to obtain required medical care
   h. Inappropriate home maintenance
3. Psychological findings include:
   a. Evidence of increased stress and more frequent crises
   b. Inappropriate coping
   c. Inappropriate expression of anger or guilt (in either the older adult or the abuser)

D. Nursing implications
   1. Assess the patient's activities on a typical day
   2. Review the patient's history for recent crises and alcohol or drug use
   3. Find out how much outside contact the patient has
   4. Evaluate the patient's perceptions of the current situation
   5. Assess the degree of the patient's physical, emotional, and financial dependency; also assess the availability of shelter from the abuser
   6. Intervene for specific health problems as identified
   7. Make appropriate referrals
      a. Community support services, such as day care, home health care, and Meals on Wheels, if necessary, to decrease stress on the abuser
      b. Counseling services for all parties
      c. Social service agencies, such as Adult Protective Services (if available)
      d. Legal services, such as Legal Aid Services and the American Civil Liberties Union
   8. Keep in mind that most states require health care personnel to report suspected cases of abuse
   9. Contact community emergency services
   10. Participate in abuse prevention activities, such as public education and anticipatory guidance for potential abusers
   11. Act as an advocate for increased resources for support activities and respite care and for legislation for mandatory reporting of abuse

II. Crime

A. General information
   1. The perception of crime incidence against older adults far exceeds the actual number of crimes committed against older adults
   2. Physical, financial, and environmental factors associated with aging increase older adults' vulnerability to crime

3. Older adults fear crime more than they fear illness or inadequate income
4. Crimes against older adults include personal and household larceny, household burglary, vehicular theft, assault, robbery, fraudulent schemes, purse snatching, pickpocketing, and rape
5. Fraudulent schemes aimed at older adults involve medical quackery, unreliable or unethical home repair persons, and unscrupulous salespersons (including insurance salespersons) and other businesspersons
6. Older adults suffer no greater physical injury or financial loss from crime than do younger persons
   a. However, the consequences of crime may be more devastating to older adults
   b. Major effects of crime on older adults are fear, isolation, loneliness, and feelings of powerlessness

B. Risk group characteristics
   1. Persons at high risk for suffering personal crime are men age 60 to 70, minorities, unmarried persons, and those with an income below $5,000
   2. Persons at high risk for suffering property crime are those age 65 to 75, minorities, and those living in large communities
   3. Income and location are more significant factors than age
   4. Persons age 40 to 65 are more likely to be injured during a criminal attack

C. Nursing implications
   1. Teach older adults to become familiar with and use available community services, such as escort services, block watch, and neighborhood protective networks, to reduce fear and isolation
   2. Be aware that the Law Enforcement Assistance Administration helps crime victims
   3. Know that crime victims can request that a representative of the Office of Community Victim Assistance Programs be present at the hospital or police station; this person also can teach older adults about crime prevention
   4. Refer older adults for crime prevention programs and community safety inspections aimed at increasing security-conscious behavior, establishing security procedures, and obtaining security devices
   5. Help older adults identify ways to decrease their vulnerability
   6. Encourage older adults to have Social Security checks mailed or wired directly to the bank to decrease the risk of mugging
   7. Act as an advocate for preventive programs, victim assistance programs, and establishment of community resources

III. Protective services

A. General information
   1. *Adult protective services* is a general term for services provided to protect an incompetent person from harm resulting from inability to provide self-care or to manage daily affairs
   2. The goal is to provide protection with minimal life-style disruption and with the least restrictive care alternatives, balancing freedom with safety
   3. In some communities, the Adult Protective Services agency offers a wide range of medical, legal, and social services
   4. Protective services needed by older adults may include:
      a. Social support
      b. Housing assistance
      c. Support with activities of daily living
      d. Legal aid
      e. Financial support
      f. Medical and personal care
      g. Emergency services
   5. Five types of protective legal arrangements exist for older adults
      a. POWER OF ATTORNEY
         (1) This is a legal device whereby an older adult designates another person to manage affairs
         (2) The older adult must be legally competent to initiate this action
      b. JOINT TENANCY, a legal device allowing either an older adult or the person having power of attorney to manage the former's affairs
      c. INTERVIVOS TRUST, a trust created by an older adult in which that person serves as first trustee and names a successor as the second trustee
      d. CONSERVATORSHIP
         (1) In this arrangement, a person or institution is designated to take over and protect the interests of a person judged to be incompetent
         (2) The court appoints a conservator after investigating the person's competence
         (3) This is the most restrictive form of protective service; the incompetent person no longer has the right to vote, manage money, determine residence, or make other major decisions
         (4) Most conservatorships are created for persons over age 75
         (5) Petition for conservatorship is made by the family or an institution
      e. INFORMAL GUARDIANSHIP, a nonlegal arrangement whereby a neighbor, nursing home, private attorney, bank, trust company, or nonprofit corporation acts as informal guardian for an older adult

6. Protective rights of older adults include:
   a. The right to make decisions, unless this responsibility has been delegated to another person voluntarily or by the court
   b. The right to choose to live in a harmful or self-destructive situation as long as the older adult is mentally competent, does not harm others, and commits no crime
7. Patients in long-term care facilities have the following rights:
   a. Contract rights
   b. Rights of association and communication
   c. Rights of autonomy, privacy, and security
   d. Rights related to admission, transfer, or discharge
   e. Civil and humanitarian rights
8. Protective rights are associated with certain problems
   a. Perception of COMPETENCY based on socioeconomic status
      (1) An affluent person whose behavior is unusual typically is perceived as eccentric
      (2) In contrast, a poor person whose behavior is unusual typically is perceived as incompetent
   b. Possibility of partial competency
      (1) A person may be competent in certain areas but incompetent to make complex decisions
      (2) Unless specific areas of competency are identified, an older adult may be perceived as totally incompetent (for instance, an older adult woman who is judged incompetent to manage her own affairs may be perceived as incompetent in all areas)
      (3) Limits of protective services are based on the degree of protection needed
   c. Common perception that informal guardianships have little benefit because of purported poor management and abuse

B. Nursing implications
   1. Assess and screen areas of patient competency carefully because assessment findings have legal, economic, and self-determination consequences
   2. Refer the patient and family for protective services, if necessary
   3. If informal guardianship has been established, make sure the patient knows which rights have been suspended and understands those rights that remain intact
   4. Report observations of the patient's capacity to manage daily affairs

IV. Informed consent

A. General information
   1. A patient must give informed consent before a procedure or treatment can be performed
      a. If the patient has been judged incompetent, a guardian must give consent

       b. An institutionalized patient has the same rights as other citizens; however, in some cases, such a patient unjustly is denied the right to consent

  2. To give valid consent, a patient must be competent and informed fully of all risks and benefits of a procedure or treatment

  3. The federal Department of Health and Human Services also mandates that informed consent be obtained and human subject review conducted before a patient can participate in research

       a. Guidelines establish informed consent procedures and monitor the risk-benefit ratio in studies using human subjects

       b. In research involving an incompetent patient, the investigator must obtain permission from the appropriate authority; such research is subject to strict review

B. Nursing implications

  1. Assess and screen areas of patient competency carefully to ensure informed consent

  2. Be aware that informed consent is required before any treatment or surgical or invasive procedure (depending on the facility, consent also may be required for other types of procedures)

  3. Follow legal requirements and specific procedures of the health care facility when obtaining the patient's consent

  4. Follow federal guidelines for consent when the patient participates in research

V. Quality of life and related ethical issues

A. General information

  1. In quality-of-life decisions, the risks of diagnostic testing and treatment are weighed against the chance of benefit and maintenance or enhancement of the quality of life

  2. Various factors affect decisions involving quality of life

       a. Advances in diagnostic techniques (for instance, echograms, scans, and cardiac catheterization)

       b. Advances in treatment (such as surgical cures, joint replacement, transplants, cryosurgery, microsurgery, chemotherapy, radiation therapy, and life-support techniques)

       c. Increased risk, cost, and in some cases questionable benefit associated with advanced techniques

       d. Increased data base for decision making because of specialization and development of science and technology

  3. Ethical issues arise in care situations in which scientific and medical goals may conflict with ethical and humanistic values; examples include the following:

       a. Whether to initiate or continue treatment of a terminally ill patient (and who should make this decision)

     b. Whether to withhold tube feedings for brain-dead patients; also, the issue of who should make this decision

     c. Whether to use costly medical treatments, such as organ transplantation, for very old patients; also, the issue of who should make this decision

B. Related considerations
1. Medical science now can prevent and cure many diseases
2. Death from organ failure can be postponed
3. Older adults have a greater incidence of heart attacks, cancer, and cerebrovascular accident than younger persons; curing one disease may not enhance the patient's quality of life if the patient has additional chronic diseases
4. Many therapies have an unknown risk-benefit ratio for older adults; reasons include the following:
     a. Usual testing of clinical treatments and research protocols on younger persons
     b. Unknown long-term survival rates of some therapies with questionable value or high risk
     c. Risk of poor tolerance of, unusual reactions to, or questionable value of certain therapies

C. Nursing implications
1. Know that the American Nurses' Association (ANA) Code of Ethics and Professional Standards provides guidelines for resolving ethical questions
2. Be aware that ethical rounds help nurses clarify issues and develop approaches to quality-of-life dilemmas
3. Use the following concepts and principles to guide ethical decision making:
     a. Autonomy (the right of individuals to make their own decisions as well as the right to information on which to base such decisions)
     b. Nonmaleficence (avoidance of inflicting harm)
     c. Beneficence (taking of actions that contribute to others' health and welfare)
     d. Justice (administration of what is fair, good, and deserved; for example, treatment that reflects human worth and dignity)
4. Keep in mind that the goal of ethical decision making is to determine which action is in the patient's best interest
5. Remember that ethical decision making takes into account multiple variables and is based on:
     a. The patient's condition and physical and psychosocial history
     b. Predicted outcome of therapies
6. Negotiate care goals with the patient
7. Support the patient's decision about care choices; also support the family and others involved in the patient's care

8. Be aware that ethical dilemmas necessitate communication with and respect for the patient and the perspectives of all team members

VI. Right to die

A. General information
1. Patients have the right to decide not to prolong life by extraordinary means
2. Advances in technology allow prolongation of life
3. The main issue is quality of life versus length of life
4. The decision regarding the right to die is an ethical and legal one; some states have right-to-die laws and legislation, such as living wills (a time-limited, patient-initiated, legal method for addressing the issue)
5. In right-to-die situations, the patient and family are involved in anticipatory discussions; the patient makes the decision after consulting with the physician and other health team members
6. When the patient is comatose or otherwise unable to make the decision, the family or the physician makes it
7. Factors that influence the decision to die include:
   a. Patient's and family's expressed wishes
   b. Degree of the patient's suffering
   c. Degree of the patient's cognitive impairment
   d. Prognosis
   e. Quality of life
   f. Current care setting
8. Supportive care continues after the involved parties decide that a patient should be allowed to die
9. Supportive care limits specific treatment and preserves the patient's dignity and comfort; it includes:
   a. Skin care
   b. Bowel and bladder management
   c. Oral hygiene
   d. Emotional comfort

B. Related considerations
1. Family members may disagree with the patient's decision
2. The patient may not be competent to make the decision
3. The decision not to resuscitate, hospitalize, or treat a patient may lead to one of the following orders:
   a. "Do not resuscitate" (DNR)
   b. "Do not hospitalize" (DNH)
   c. "Do not treat" (DNT)
4. A physician's signature is required for DNR, DNH, and DNT orders
5. DNR, DNH, and DNT orders are used more frequently in nursing homes than in hospitals
6. Legal protection is provided only when physicians and health care facilities follow appropriate policies and procedures

7. EUTHANASIA may take one of two forms
    a. Active euthanasia, in which another person helps someone die
    b. Passive euthanasia, in which a person is permitted to die through another person's refusal to interfere actively with natural processes

C. Nursing implications
    1. Support the patient and family in decision making
    2. Support nurses and physicians who implement right-to-die policies
    3. Ensure that supportive care is maintained after the decision is made

Points to remember

In most states, health care workers must report suspected cases of abuse.

Major effects of crime on older adults are fear, isolation, loneliness, and feelings of powerlessness.

A conservatorship is the most restrictive form of protective service.

Determining a client's competency status and functional abilities has legal, economic, and self-determination consequences.

Glossary

The following terms are defined in Appendix A, page 194.

abuse	intervivos trust
competency	joint tenancy
conservatorship	neglect
euthanasia	power of attorney
informal guardianship	

Study questions

To evaluate your understanding of this chapter, answer the following questions in the space provided; then compare your responses with the correct answers in Appendix B, page 206.

1. What are three behavioral findings that suggest abuse in an older adult?

_____

_____

2. What is a conservatorship? _____

_____

3. Which criteria are necessary for a person to give valid consent? _____

_____

_____

4. What are some appropriate nursing actions to take when a patient decides not to prolong life by extraordinary means? _____

_____

CHAPTER 10

Economics and Health Care

Learning objectives

Check off the following items once you've mastered them:

☐ Identify special concerns that older adults may have regarding work and retirement.

☐ Name Social Security Administration programs that provide income and health care for poor older adults.

☐ State major sources of income for older adults.

☐ Identify the differences between Medicare part A and Medicare part B.

I. Older adults and the economy

A. General information
1. Various factors influence the economy
   a. Demographic changes
   b. Social and economic policies affecting older adults' choices about retirement
   c. Changes in retirement patterns (which affect the Social Security Administration's deficit)
2. Problems in financing social welfare programs stem from various causes
   a. Changes in economic conditions
   b. Higher unemployment rates
   c. Rapid inflation
   d. Lower productivity

B. Economic resources for older adults
1. Public financing comes from taxation
2. Private income and savings are a major economic resource

II. Work and retirement

A. Aging of the work force
1. The work force now includes a higher proportion of older adults
2. Older adults who stay in the same positions limit other workers' movement into entry positions and upward mobility
3. In 1978, the Amendment to Age Discrimination in Employment Act raised the mandatory retirement age from 65 to 70
4. In 1989, more than 50% of older adult workers were part-time employees
5. In 1989, 12% of older adults were in the labor force
6. In 1989, older adults accounted for less than 3% of the labor force
   a. Three of every five persons in this group were between ages 65 and 69
   b. 14% were over age 75

B. Retirement age
1. The age at which older adults retire affects the work force
   a. More people are retiring earlier and living longer
   b. Factors affecting older adults' ability to retain employment include age discrimination, potentially reduced competence, job "burnout," and physiologic decline
2. Private pension plans may include written provisions that encourage early retirement

C. Decrease in income
1. Inflation makes saving for retirement difficult
2. Income typically decreases after retirement

III. Post-retirement income

A. Government income maintenance policies
1. Social Security
   a. Social Security legislation was enacted in 1935
   b. This law provides for a continuing income when a person's job earnings stop or decrease from retirement, disability, or a spouse's death
   c. Eligibility is based on work credits earned under Social Security
   d. Social Security benefits come from Social Security taxes paid by employees, employers, and self-employed workers
   e. Benefits are based on the amount the worker paid from earnings over a period of years; a government formula determines the amount of the benefit
   f. Benefits include retirement checks (when an worker retires), disability checks (when a worker becomes seriously disabled), and survivor's checks (which go to certain family members when a worker dies)
   g. Benefits also are paid to certain dependents of workers who have retired, become disabled, or died
   h. Benefits periodically are adjusted for inflation
   i. Benefits are intended to provide income protection, not to replace all lost earnings
   j. Ideally, retirement income should include a combination of Social Security benefits, pensions, investments, private savings, and income from other sources
2. Welfare programs
   a. Government welfare programs benefit many older adults, helping to ensure that they maintain a predetermined standard of living
   b. Eligibility is based on economic status, not age
      (1) To be eligible, a person must have income and assets that fall below specified levels
      (2) Blind persons, disabled persons, older adults, and mothers with dependent children usually are eligible
   c. Supplemental Security Income (SSI) ensures a minimum monthly income to needy persons with limited income who are blind, disabled, or elderly
      (1) SSI is a federal program administered by states; SSI programs include food stamps, social services programs, and Medicaid programs
      (2) Eligibility for food stamps varies from state to state
      (3) Social services programs were initiated through the Older Americans Act of 1965, which authorized funding for services to older adults
         (a) These programs emphasize maintaining older adults in the community

(b) Funds are channeled to states, communities, and nonprofit organizations (through the Administration on Aging)

(c) Channeling of services through state and area agencies helps coordinate delivery of services in the community

(d) Information about Administration on Aging services is available at local agencies on aging

(4) MEDICAID was established by Title 19 of the Social Security Act

(a) It is a joint federal-state program that pays physician bills, hospital bills, nursing home bills, and other related health care costs of eligible poor persons

(b) Eligibility requirements vary from state to state

3. Pensions

a. Pensions provide income for many older adults

b. Pension regulations have been established by the federal government

c. Retirement savings get preferential tax treatment

d. Pension funds must be insured by the Pension Benefit Guarantee Corporation (U.S. Department of Labor) to protect against employer bankruptcy and to qualify for tax breaks

e. The employee Retirement Income Security Act of 1974 required employers to establish vesting standards

f. The federal Civil Service Retirement System includes executive, judicial, and legislative government employees

g. Separate retirement pension systems exist for employees of the Federal Reserve System and Tennessee Valley Authority and members of the armed forces

h. Most states have separate retirement pension systems for state and local government employees

B. Personal income and economic status of older adults

1. Sources of income

a. Older adults derive income from Social Security benefits, asset income, earnings, public and private pensions, and other sources

b. Social Security benefits are the major source of income for older adults; for approximately 20% of older adults, Social Security benefits are the sole source of income

c. Benefits from MEDICARE, Medicaid, housing assistance, and food stamp programs can increase a single person's income by 32% and a family's income by 14%

d. Purchasing power is affected by personal wealth, continued earnings, government funds, and family assistance

2. Economic status

a. The economic status of older adults has improved significantly over the last 20 years

(1) A gain in earnings has led to increased savings

(2) This, in turn, has increased post-retirement income
  b. For female heads of household age 65 or older, the median income increased from $3,514 in 1959 to $12,881 in 1980; this represents a 40% increase in real income
  c. The number of older adults with incomes below the poverty level fell from 5.5 million in 1959 to 3.4 million in 1989

IV. Health care utilization and costs

A. Use of health care services
  1. Older adults are heavy users of health care services
    a. 33% of all hospitalized patients are older adults
    b. In 1987, older adults accounted for 36% of total personal health care expenditures
    c. In 1988, older adults accounted for 44% of all hospital days
  2. The average length of hospital stay of older adults is 8 to 9 days
  3. Older adults average nine physician visits per year

B. Health care costs of older adults
  1. In 1987, health care costs for older adults averaged $5,360
  2. Hospital expenses account for 42% of older adults' health care costs
  3. Physician bills account for about 21% of older adults' health care costs
  4. Nursing home expenses account for roughly 20% of older adults' health care costs
  5. In 1987, 63% of health care costs were covered by government programs (government-calculated health care costs do not include the cost of assistance from families)

V. Health care system and the health problems of older adults

A. Premise and focus of health care policy
  1. Health care policy in the United States assumes that health care is a personal responsibility
  2. The U.S. health care system and health care resources are organized to manage specialty acute-care problems, not chronic, degenerative, multiple health problems
  3. However, the health problems of older adults are chronic, degenerative, and multiple

B. Continuity of care and health promotion
  1. Continuity of care between hospitals and community-based primary and rehabilitative care facilities is poor, at best; in some cases, it is nonexistent
  2. Health promotion and illness prevention may or may not help lower the incidence or delay the onset of chronic disease or reduce the degree of disability

VI. Medicare reimbursement

A. Medicare part A
1. This program was established by the federal government in 1965 to assist older adults with health care costs
2. It covers inpatient hospital care, medically necessary inpatient care in a SKILLED NURSING FACILITY (SNF) after a hospital stay, home health care, and HOSPICE care
3. Peer Review Organizations (PROs), which consist of a group of physicians, are paid by the federal government to review Medicare-related hospital care and to investigate patient complaints
4. Eligibility for Medicare part A is based on the patient's Social Security work record or federal employment
5. Benefits are paid on the basis of benefit periods
   a. The benefit period begins on the first day the patient receives Medicare-covered services and ends when the patient has remained out of the hospital or SNF for 60 consecutive days
   b. Admission to a hospital after 60 days begins a new benefit period
   c. The number of benefit periods for a hospital or skilled nursing facility is unlimited
   d. Special limited benefit periods apply to hospice care
6. Medicare part A covers most, but not all, services
   a. It pays for all covered services for the first 60 days of inpatient hospital care in the benefit period (except a deductible – $592 in 1990)
   b. For the next 30 days, it pays for all covered services, except $148 per day (in 1990)
   c. If a patient needs more than 90 days of coverage in a given benefit period, 60 reserve days are available
      (1) Medicare Part A covers all but $296 per day (in 1990)
      (2) Reserve days are not renewable
7. Medicare part A covers SNF care for skilled nursing and rehabilitation services
   a. The SNF must be Medicare-certified
   b. As of 1990, Medicare part A pays for all covered services for the first 20 days and pays all costs except $74 per day for the next 80 days
8. Medicare part A covers medically necessary home health services
   a. It covers the cost of a part-time visiting nurse and physical or speech therapist from a Medicare-certified home health agency
   b. It may cover the cost of part-time home health aide services, occupational therapy, medical services, and medical supplies
9. Hospice care is covered under Medicare part A for a maximum of two 90-day benefit periods and one 30-day benefit period; no deductibles or copayments are involved except for outpatient drugs and inpatient respite care

10. The prospective payment system requires hospitals to accept Medicare payment as payment in full and prohibits hospitals from billing patients for anything except applicable deductible and coinsurance amounts plus services and items not covered (such as private television, private duty nurse, and custodial care)

B. Medicare part B
1. This program is a voluntary medical insurance plan; the insured party pays a monthly premium
2. Medicare part B covers physician's services, excluding routine physical examinations; outpatient hospital care; home health care, if medically necessary; physical and speech therapy; and other medically necessary medical services and supplies
3. Payments are based on what the law defines as reasonable charges, not on current charges of suppliers (persons or organizations, other than physicians or health care facilities, that provide equipment or services covered by medical insurance)
4. As of 1990, the patient pays $75 of approved charges; after that, Medicare part B pays 80% of approved charges and the patient pays the remaining 20%
5. A physician, medical supplier, or therapist who accepts assignment of Medicare benefits must accept Medicare's approved amount as full payment and legally cannot bill the patient for anything over that amount
6. Physicians and suppliers who agree to accept assignment on all Medicare claims are listed in the Medicare Participating Physician Supplier Directory, available at local Social Security and Railroad Retirement Board offices and at all state and area offices of Administration on Aging

C. Some expenses not covered by Medicare parts A or B
1. Private duty nursing
2. Skilled nursing care beyond that covered by Medicare part A
3. Routine physical examinations
4. Custodial care
5. Eye or hearing examinations to prescribe or fit eyeglasses or hearing aids
6. Immunizations, except for pneumococcal vaccinations or other immunizations necessitated by injury or immediate risk of infection
7. Drugs, other than prescription drugs furnished during a stay in a hospital or SNF or provided by a hospice for symptom management
8. Dental care
9. Full-time nursing care at home

D. Payments
1. Medicare benefits change from year to year

2. The form titled "Patient's Request for Medicare Payment" (Form 14905) must be submitted to the Medicare carrier for payment
   a. A physician or supplier who uses the assignment method of payment or who is Medicare-participating submits the claim
   b. If the physician does not accept Medicare assignment, the patient submits the claim
   c. When submitting a claim for rental or purchase of durable medical equipment, the patient must include the bill from the supplier and the physician's prescription indicating the type of equipment needed, the medical reason, and estimated length of time the equipment will be medically necessary
3. Before Medicare payments are made, the patient must meet the deductible requirement
4. The billing system may be confusing to older adults, who may fear mishandling bills and checks and may have difficulty dealing with the system

VII. Private health insurance

A. General information
   1. Individual and group health insurance policies are available
   2. Coverage varies widely
   3. The value and type of private health insurance should be evaluated on an individual basis
   4. Medicaid-eligible older adults usually do not need private health insurance

B. Types of individual and group health insurance
   1. *Medicare supplementary programs* usually follow Medicare guidelines for services determined to be medically necessary
      a. These programs may pay some or all Medicare deductibles and copayments
      b. They may not be in the best interests of older adults because of their high cost and limited benefits
   2. *Catastrophic or major medical expense coverage* helps cover the cost of serious illness or injury; it includes services not covered by Medicare
   3. HEALTH MAINTENANCE ORGANIZATIONS (HMOs) charge a membership fee or premium
      a. Patients must receive services directly from HMO-affiliated physicians and other providers
      b. Health care services are prepaid
   4. *Employer group insurance* is employer-continued or conversion group insurance
   5. *Association group insurance* is obtained from organizations (other than employers) that offer various types of group health insurance for members over age 65

VIII. Nursing implications

A. Recognize the cost constraints of older adults' income restrictions

B. Plan care to contain costs; for example, recommend generic medications, community resources, and family resources

C. Become familiar with current Medicare and Medicaid requirements and limitations of service

D. Become familiar with community resources

E. Provide information and direction to help older adults contact appropriate agencies

F. Caution older adults who are considering a Medicare supplement (often called Medi-gap) to investigate the program thoroughly; some supplement programs may not be beneficial

Points to remember

Economic resources for older adults derive from taxation (public financing) and private income and savings.

Medicare part A covers hospital expenses.

Medicare part B is a voluntary medical insurance program.

Medicaid is a state-regulated medical assistance program for low-income persons.

Older adults may need help in understanding the Medicare reimbursement system.

SSI ensures a minimum monthly income to needy persons with limited income who are blind, disabled, or elderly.

Glossary

The following terms are defined in Appendix A, page 194.

health maintenance organization

hospice

Medicaid

Medicare

skilled nursing facility

Study questions

To evaluate your understanding of this chapter, answer the following questions in the space provided; then compare your responses with the correct answers in Appendix B, pages 206 and 207.

1. What are two factors that contribute to problems in financing social welfare programs? _____

   _____

2. What did the Amendment to Age Discrimination in Employment Act of 1978 accomplish? _____

   _____

3. What is the basis for determining whether a person is eligible for receiving assistance from welfare programs? _____

   _____

4. Hospital expenses account for approximately what percentage of the health care costs of older adults? _____

   _____

5. Which expenses does Medicare part A cover? _____

   _____

6. What are three types of private health insurance available to older adults?

   _____

   _____

7. What are some ways in which the nurse can help older adults deal with the economic aspects of health care? _____

   _____

CHAPTER 11

The Nurse's Role and Function in Gerontology

Learning objectives

Check off the following items once you've mastered them:

☐ Name the American Nurses' Association (ANA) document that serves as the standard for nursing practice in the care of older adults.

☐ List the seven ANA standards for gerontologic care.

☐ Define the nurse's role as advocate for older adults.

☐ Identify changes in health care delivery that may affect the gerontologic nursing role.

I. Gerontologic nursing roles and care approach

A. Nursing roles
  1. Gerontologic nursing roles include communicator, planner, case finder, caregiver, comforter, teacher, rehabilitator, and coordinator
  2. Nurses have an opportunity to provide leadership and act as agents for change in altering staff, institutional, and public policy perceptions about aging and older adults' health needs

B. Care approach
  1. Health care for older adults typically requires a multidisciplinary approach
  2. The opportunity exists for challenge and creativity in designing ways to provide quality care for older adults

II. Practice settings and focus of care

A. Practice settings
  1. The gerontologic nurse may practice in an acute-care, long-term care, or community setting
     a. Older adults occupy more than one-half of all hospital beds
     b. Older adults use approximately 60% of all health services
  2. Employment opportunities are growing in home health care agencies, WELLNESS CLINICS, and nursing homes
  3. Specialization is needed in such fields as GEROPSYCHIATRY, long-term care, and education
  4. Gerontologic knowledge also is needed in other specialties, such as oncology and rheumatology

B. Focus of care
  1. Gerontologic nursing practice may focus on elderly patients only
  2. Alternatively, it may involve a mixed caseload

III. ANA standards of gerontologic nursing practice

A. Development of standards
  1. The Division of Geriatric Nursing Practice was the first ANA specialty division to establish standards
  2. The seven standards, issued in 1969, were most recently revised in 1987 (see *ANA Standards of Gerontological Nursing Practice*, page 188)

B. Purpose of standards
  1. The ANA standards address the nursing process
  2. They emphasize active involvement by older adults in decision making and goal setting for nursing care
  3. Gerontologic nursing functions include teaching and supervising health maintenance and maximizing the patient's biological, psychological, and social resources

A.N.A. STANDARDS OF GERONTOLOGICAL NURSING PRACTICE

STANDARD I. Organization of Gerontological Nursing Services
All gerontological nursing services are planned, organized, and directed by a nurse executive. The nurse executive has baccalaureate or master's preparation and has experience in gerontological nursing and administration of long-term care services or acute care services for older clients.

STANDARD II. Theory
The nurse participates in the generation and testing of theory as a basis for clinical decisions. The nurse uses theoretical concepts to guide the effective practice of gerontological nursing.

STANDARD III. Data Collection
The health status of the older person is regularly assessed in a comprehensive, accurate, and systematic manner. The information obtained during the health assessment is accessible to and shared with appropriate members of the interdisciplinary health care team, including the older person and the family.

STANDARD IV. Nursing Diagnosis
The nurse uses health assessment data to determine nursing diagnoses.

STANDARD V. Planning and Continuity of Care
The nurse develops the plan of care in conjunction with the older person and appropriate others; mutual goals, priorities, nursing approaches, and measures in the care plan address the therapeutic, preventive, restorative, and rehabilitative needs of the older person. The care plan helps the older person attain and maintain the highest level of health, well-being, and quality of life achievable, as well as a peaceful death. The plan of care facilitates continuity of care over time as the client moves to various care settings, and is revised as necessary.

STANDARD VI. Intervention
The nurse, guided by the plan of care, intervenes to provide care to restore the older person's functional capabilities and to prevent complications and excess disability. Nursing interventions are derived from nursing diagnoses and are based on gerontological nursing theory.

STANDARD VII. Evaluation
The nurse continually evaluates the client's and family's responses to interventions in order to determine progress toward goal attainment and to revise the data base, nursing diagnoses, and plan of care.

STANDARD VIII. Interdisciplinary Collaboration
The nurse collaborates with other members of the health care team in the various settings in which care is given to the older person. The team meets regularly to evaluate the effectiveness of the care plan for the client and family and to adjust the plan of care to accommodate changing needs.

STANDARD IX. Research
The nurse participates in research designed to generate an organized body of gerontological nursing knowledge, disseminates research findings, and uses them in practice.

STANDARD X. Ethics
The nurse uses the code for nurses established by the American Nurses' Association as a guide for ethical decision making and practice.

STANDARD XI. Professional Development
The nurse assumes responsbility for professional development and contributes to the professional growth of interdisciplinary team members. The nurse participates in peer review and other means of evaluation to assure the quality of nursing practice.

From *Standards and Scope of Gerontological Nursing Practice*. Kansas City: American Nurses' Association, 1987. Used with permission.

C. Terminology change
   1. In 1975, ANA changed the term used to describe nursing for older adults from *geriatric nursing* to *gerontological nursing*
   2. Gerontologic nursing denotes care and treatment of older adults from a holistic standpoint, not just as diseased or sick persons; in contrast, geriatric nursing focuses on care of sick persons

IV. Education and certification

A. Education
   1. Undergraduate programs incorporate gerontologic components into basic nursing education
   2. Graduate programs prepare the nurse to function as a gerontologic nurse or a gerontologic nurse practitioner

B. Certification
   1. ANA administers certification examinations for gerontologic nurse and gerontologic nurse practitioner (GNP)
      a. Certification is a voluntary program
      b. The purpose of certification is to acknowledge professional achievement in nursing
      c. Certification recognizes the nurse's expertise in applying current knowledge
   2. The gerontologic nurse is responsible for assessing, planning, and implementing health care for older adults and evaluating effectiveness of care
      a. A baccalaureate degree is required
      b. Two years of clinical experience also are required
   3. The gerontologic nurse practitioner can manage 80% to 90% of care problems in nursing homes; the GNP is responsible for patient assessment and evaluation, certain diagnostic procedures, medical management according to protocol, and family assessment
      a. To become a certified gerontologic nurse practitioner, a nurse must pass a certification examination and be prepared in a nurse practitioner educational program to deliver primary health services to older adults
      b. A master's degree and practice experience are required

V. Gerontologic nursing functions

A. Acute care
   1. Obtain the patient's medical, family, and psychosocial history
   2. Perform a patient assessment
   3. Explain diagnosis and treatment to the patient and family
   4. Work closely with the patient, family, and other health professionals to develop a nursing care plan
   5. Foster the patient's independence

6. Maintain hydration, nutrition, aeration, and comfort
7. Provide prescribed medications and treatment; evaluate the patient's response
8. Inform the physician of any change in the patient's condition
9. Administer emergency treatments when necessary
10. Initiate discharge planning and coordinate referrals to appropriate community agencies
11. Serve as patient advocate

B. Long-term care
1. Obtain the patient's medical, family, and psychosocial history
2. Perform a patient assessment
3. Involve the patient and family in preparing and implementing the care plan
4. Promote an atmosphere that emphasizes living, not disease and dying
5. Ensure that the patient receives appropriate medical, dental, and podiatric care
6. Maintain hydration, nutrition, aeration, and comfort
7. Provide prescribed medications, treatments, and rehabilitative exercises; evaluate the patient's response
8. Inform the physician of any change in the patient's condition
9. Perform emergency measures when necessary
10. Teach and advise the patient and family about the disease and its management
11. Become familiar with community services for older adults and refer the patient and family to such services, as appropriate
12. Serve as patient advocate

C. Community care
1. Identify the patient's health, social, and economic needs
2. Provide referrals to the health professional or agency best able to meet the patient's needs
3. Explain diagnosis and treatment to the patient and family
4. Evaluate the patient's compliance with and response to treatment
5. Use clinic and home visits for health promotion
6. Teach and advise the patient and family about the disease and its management
7. Evaluate the patient's ability to live independently
8. Act as an advocate for older adults
9. Encourage older adults to become advocates on their own behalf

VI. Issues affecting gerontologic nursing roles

A. Gerontologic nursing research
1. Nursing studies develop gerontologic knowledge by recognizing problems and asking questions; all nurses can participate in such studies

2. Nursing studies on clinical problems are needed to improve the quality of care for older adults
3. Research areas include cognitive function, nutrition, demographic changes, epidemiology, life-style changes, wellness behaviors, sleep patterns, and skin care problems
4. Research also is needed on how to adapt or change nursing interventions for older adults

B. Advocacy
   1. Advocacy refers to representing the interests of another person or group to influence institutional, administrative, or legislative policy
      a. The purpose is to ensure equal opportunity and obtain services that the person or group has been unable to obtain
      b. Most definitions of a nurse include the advocacy role
   2. Advocacy is a dynamic process
      a. The nurse-advocate assumes an active, assertive role as an agent for change
      b. Issues appropriate for advocacy may include human rights and responsibilities, ethics, and self-determination
      c. The advocacy role may include providing support, sharing information, and working through political channels to benefit older adults
      d. Nurses need to become active in gerontologic nursing organizations, such as ANA's Council on Gerontological Nursing, to help effect change

C. Changes in health care delivery
   1. The prospective payment system for health care costs, implementation of DIAGNOSTIC-RELATED GROUPS (DRGs), and the trend toward early discharge have increased the number of older adults needing community services
   2. Because more advanced technological equipment, such as respirators and feeding pumps, can be used at home, many patients now leave the hospital sooner
   3. Development of a prospective payment system for nursing homes and community care may be implemented

D. Development of ANA councils, such as the Council on Gerontological Nursing, to set standards

E. Movement of practitioner education into graduate nursing programs

F. Efforts to obtain third-party reimbursement for nurse practitioners

G. Demonstration projects, such as TEACHING NURSING HOMES

Points to remember

The gerontologic nurse may practice in an acute care, long-term care, or community setting.

The ANA has established standards of gerontologic nursing practice.

Gerontologic clinical research is needed to improve the quality of care.

Advocacy, a nursing role, involves representing the interests of another person or a group.

Glossary

The following terms are defined in Appendix A, page 194.

diagnostic-related groups

geropsychiatry

teaching nursing home

wellness clinic

Study questions

To evaluate your understanding of this chapter, answer the following questions in the space provided; then compare your responses with the correct answers in Appendix B, page 207.

1. What are three roles of the gerontologic nurse? _____

   _____

2. How does gerontologic nursing differ from geriatric nursing? _____

   _____

   _____

3. What are the requirements for certification as a gerontologic nurse practi-

   tioner? _____

   _____

4. What are three gerontologic nursing functions in community care?

   _____

   _____

5. What are two issues affecting the gerontologic nursing role? _____

   _____

   _____

Appendices

A: Glossary

Abuse – misuse or maltreatment that places a person in jeopardy

Ageism – attitudinal prejudice against older persons

Aging – normal, universal, progressive, irreversible process that occurs with passage of time

Antibody – immunoglobulin produced in response to an antigen

Antigen – substance that elicits an immunologic response

Aphasia – abnormal neurologic condition causing a defect in receptive or expressive language function (speech)

Apraxia – inability to perform purposeful acts or manipulate objects

Arcus senilis – glossy white line that completely or partially encircles the periphery of the iris

Arteriosclerosis obliterans – condition involving occlusion of an artery of the lower extremities resulting in tissue ischemia

Astereognosis – inability to identify objects by touch

Claudication – complaint of pain in an extremity when walking which subsides with rest.

Cohort – group of persons having a demographic factor in common (such as being born in a given year or period) who have experienced the same life events and who share a similar view of the world

Competency – ability to perform certain acts, determine right and wrong, make decisions, and take responsibility for them

Conductive hearing loss – hearing loss that results from an impediment in the mechanical transmission of sound from the external ear through to the inner ear; sound intensity is diminished but clarity is unchanged

Congregate meals—provision of a nutritionally balanced meal to a group of persons, usually older adults, at the same time

Conservatorship—arrangement whereby a person or institution is appointed by the court to take over and protect the interests of a person judged to be incompetent; the most restrictive form of protective service

Creatinine—end product of creatine metabolism commonly found in the blood and muscle tissue; filtered by the kidneys and excreted in urine

Crepitus—crackling sound similar to that of rubbing hair between fingers, associated with gas gangrene or rubbing of bone fragments

Crystallized intelligence—cognitive processes and abilities developed through the context of cultural meaning, (mainly education and life experience); uses experience as a problem-solving base

Cystocele—prolapse of the bladder wall into the vagina

Death-denying—refusing to recognize death as a natural part of existence

Delirium—acute organic mental disorder evidenced by confusion, disorientation, restlessness, and clouded sensorium

Dementia—deterioration or loss of intellectual faculties, reasoning power, and memory

Diagnostic-related group—designation used to set predetermined Medicare reimbursement rates based on classification by patient diagnosis rather than on charges accumulated during length of stay

Diplopia—double vision

Drug absorption—passage of a drug across and into tissues

Drug distribution—movement of an absorbed drug from the systemic circulation into organs and peripheral tissues

Drug excretion—process by which a substance (such as a drug) is eliminated from the body

Drug metabolism—sum of all chemical reactions involved in the biotransformation of a drug

Dysarthria—speech that is poorly articulated because of a defect in the muscles of speech

Dysphagia — difficulty in swallowing

Dysphasia — difficulty speaking

Ego integrity — acknowledgment or awareness that life has value and purpose and the self is complete

Eschar — scarred, dry crusted tissue resulting usually from a burn, infection, or excoriating skin disease

Euthanasia — active or passive act of permitting or bringing about death in a relatively painless way in a person suffering from a painful, incurable disease

Exophthalmos — marked protrusion of the eyeballs

Fluid intelligence — cognitive processes and abilities relating to neurophysiologic status; creates innovative behavior

Free radical — molecule with an extra electric charge, having a free electron

Functional ability — ability to perform physical and instrumental activities of daily living

Functional assessment — type of assessment that measures a patient's overall well-being and self-care abilities

Functional reserve — body's ability to adapt to changes

Geriatrics — study of the diseases of aging

Gerontology — study of all aspects and problems of aging, including physiologic, pathologic, psychological, economic, and sociologic

Geropsychiatry — branch of medicine that deals with the study, treatment, and prevention of mental disorders in older adult persons

Glomerular filtration rate — amount of plasma filtrate that passes through the glomeruli of both kidneys each minute

Health maintenance organization — private health insurance that provides basic and supplemental health services (including preventive care and treatment) to members who prepay a fixed periodic fee

Hemianopia — loss of vision in half the visual field (usually the vertical half) of one or both eyes

Hemiplegia — paralysis of one side of the body

Homeostasis — balance of the body's internal environment

Homonymous hemianopia — defective vision in right or left halves of the visual field of both eyes

Hospice — multidisciplinary system of patient care designed to assist the terminally ill patient and family to be comfortable and to maintain a satisfactory life-style through the phases of dying

Hyperemia — increased circulation of blood to an area, manifested by redness and increased temperature of that area

Hypertonia — excessive muscular contraction resulting from continuous nerve stimulation

Hyphema — hemorrhage into the anterior chamber of the eye

Informal guardianship — nonlegal arrangement in which another party (such as a neighbor, nursing home, private attorney, bank, trust company, or nonprofit corporation) acts as guardian for an older adult

Instrumental ADLS — activities that involve task performance at a higher level focusing on the patient's ability to interact with the environment, such as telephoning, shopping, preparing meals, cleaning, taking medication, and managing finances

Intermediate-care facility — facility that provides custodial care and personal-care services to patients requiring less than 24-hour-a-day nursing care

Intervivos trust — trust created by an older adult in which that person serves as first trustee and names a successor as the second trustee

Ischemia — decreased blood supply to a body part

Joint tenancy — legal device that allows either an older adult or a person having power of attorney for an older adult to manage the former's affairs

Kegel exercise — exercise that strengthens perineal muscles

Leukoplakia — precancerous condition characterized by white spots or patches on the mucous membrane of the tongue or cheek

Long-term memory — storage of information (large amounts) whose recall can be delayed for long periods of time

Medicaid — federally funded, state-operated medical assistance program for low-income persons

Medicare — federally funded health maintenance program for persons age 65 or older

Miosis — pupillary constriction

Miotic — agent that constricts the pupils

Mydriatic — agent that dilates the pupils

Neglect — failure to give proper care or attention

Net worth — assets minus liabilities

Neurogenic incontinence — involuntary discharge of urine caused by alteration in the sensory and motor tracts involved in bladder muscle function

Older adult — adult age 65 or over

Old-old adult — adult between ages 80 and 99

Orthopnea — condition requiring the person to sit or stand in order to breathe comfortably

Overflow incontinence — dribbling of urine resulting from an obstructive lesion or drug-induced urine retention

Paraphasia — use of incorrect words when speaking

Paresis — partial paralysis

Paresthesia — abnormal sensations, such as numbness or tingling

Peak experience — experience that transcends ordinary limitations and experiences

Phacoemulsification — fragmentation of the lens of the eye by ultrasonic vibrations, with simultaneous irrigation and aspiration; a treatment for cataracts

Polydipsia — excessive thirst

Polyphagia – excessive eating

Polypharmacy – the administration of many drugs together or the administration of excessive medication

Polyuria – excessive urination

Power of attorney – legal device whereby a legally competent older adult designates another person to manage affairs

Presbycusis – age-related hearing change involving decreases in hearing acuity, auditory threshold, pitch and tone discrimination, and ability to understand speech

Presbyopia – age-related vision change characterized by decreased ability of the eye to accommodate for close work

Primary memory – memory that consists of information held in temporary storage for active processing

Proprioception – sensation of body position, movement, and equilibrium, transmitted from specialized nerve endings located mainly in muscles, tendons, and the labyrinth of the inner ear

Protective environment – setting that provides safety and security for an older adult or other person

Pulse pressure – numerical difference between systolic blood pressure and diastolic blood pressure; normally 30 to 40 mm Hg

Respite care – short-term care of an older adult or other patient intended to give family caregivers a rest

Reticular activating system – functional brain system responsible for wakefulness, attention, concentration, and introspection

Secondary memory – memory consisting of information that is held in storage and must be retrieved

Senile purpura – bruises appearing just under the skin of elderly persons

Sensorineural hearing loss – failure in transmission of sound within inner ear or brain because of impaired cochlea or 8th cranial nerve function

Short-term memory — memory encompassing components of both primary and secondary memory and available for instantaneous use

Skilled nursing facility — specially qualified facility with staff and equipment needed to provide skilled nursing care or rehabilitative services

Sleep apnea — temporary cessation of breathing during sleep

Somatic mutation — failure or error in the replication of deoxyribonucleic acid

Stenosis — narrowing or constriction of an opening or passageway

Stress incontinence — involuntary discharge of urine with increased abdominal pressure; typically occurs during sneezing, coughing, or laughing

Teaching nursing home — nursing home linked with an educational institution for instruction of students and training of physicians and nurses in gerontologic care

Urgency incontinence — involuntary discharge of large amounts of urine after a sudden urge to void

Uveitis — inflammation of the iris, ciliary body, and choroid (uveal tract) of the eye

Valsalva maneuver — forced expiratory effort against a closed glottis, such as when a person holds the breath and tenses the muscles in an effort to change position in bed; causes an increase in intrathoracic pressure, which in turn decreases venous return to the right side of the heart

Wellness clinic — clinic that specializes in health promotion and maintenance

Young-old adult — adult between ages 60 and 79

B: Answers to Study Questions

CHAPTER 1

1. Two factors affecting the age distribution of the population are decreased mortality and decreased fertility.

2. Alaska, Nevada, Hawaii, Arizona, New Mexico, South Carolina, Utah, Florida, North Carolina, and Delaware had more than 10% growth in the older adult population between 1980 and 1989.

3. Sources of income for older adults include Social Security, asset income, earnings, pensions, and Supplemental Security Income.

4. Most older adults rate their health as good or excellent compared with others their age.

5. The two leading causes of death in older adults are heart disease and cancer.

6. The fastest growing segment of the older adult population is over age 75.

CHAPTER 2

1. Three characteristics that theories of aging must include are a description of aging as universal in all species members; a description of aging as progressive over the life span; and a description of aging as debilitative, leading to degenerative changes and failure of systems.

2. Intrinsic biological theories maintain that aging changes arise from internal, predetermined causes; extrinsic biological theories maintain that aging results from environmental factors that cause changes in the body.

3. Psychological theories attempt to explain aging changes in cognitive functions, such as intelligence, memory, learning, and problem solving.

4. The activity theory proposes that successful aging depends on maintaining a high level of activity and that involvement in life is associated with life satisfaction.

CHAPTER 3

1. Factors to assess when evaluating the older adult's adjustment to aging include self-image, growth and self-actualization, integration of personality, autonomy, realistic perception of the self and world, and environmental mastery.

2. Developmental tasks described by Robert Peck include ego differentiation vs. work-role preoccupation, body transcendence vs. body preoccupation, and ego transcendence vs. ego preoccupation.

3. Factors associated with role adjustment include (any three) age, sex, culture, beliefs, attitudes, income, health, and past experiences.

4. Stereotypical attitudes can affect health care workers in all aspects of care planning and implementation, career choice and job selection, salaries, and policy and program development.

5. The nurse should support the older adult's religious beliefs and practices, find out what the patient wants, and not assume that the patient desires religious consultation or participation in services. The nurse also should keep in mind that spiritual well-being is as important as physical and psychological well-being.

CHAPTER 4

1. By age 75, body fat increases and body water decreases.

2. With age, cellular turnover diminishes (from slow cell reproduction in the epidermis and dermis), blood supply and subcutaneous fat decrease, and skin becomes thinner.

3. The number and size of pulmonary alveoli decrease with age.

4. Age-related electrocardiogram changes include increased P-R, QRS, and Q-T intervals; decreased amplitude of the QRS complex; and a leftward shift of the QRS axis.

5. Accumulation of fat tissue in the stomach causes delayed gastric emptying and difficulty in managing large food quantities.

6. The glomerular filtration rate (GFR) starts to decline at about age 40.

7. With age, monoamine oxidase and serotonin levels increase and norepinephrine and dopamine levels decrease.

8. Glucose tolerance decreases with age.

9. Bone loss and decreased water content of intervertebral disks contribute to height reduction.

CHAPTER 5

1. Nursing goals for the patient with delirium include establishing a meaningful environment; helping to maintain body awareness; and helping the patient cope with confusion and any hallucinations, delusions, or illusions.

2. In an older adult with chronic arterial insufficiency, the nurse should assess for an ulcer with well-defined edges, black or necrotic tissue, a deep base, pale color, and no bleeding.

3. Arrhythmias are more serious in older adults than in younger adults because of their lower tolerance for decreased cardiac output, which can lead to syncope, falls, transient ischemic attacks, and possible dementia.

4. In a patient with cataracts, the nurse should expect poor vision; eye fatigue; headache; increased light sensitivity; blurred or multiple vision; and difficulty coping with sudden darkness, bright lights, and glare.

5. In a patient with left-sided hemiplegia, the nurse should expect dysarthria (which may result from impaired coordination of speech muscles, such as from nerve damage) and difficulty speaking clearly. Typically, this patient does not have trouble choosing words or understanding speech.

6. Nursing goals for older adults with congestive heart failure (CHF) include decreasing the cardiac workload, increasing cardiac output, and reducing vascular congestion.

7. Factors that place older adults at increased risk for decubitus ulcers include (any three) immobility; impaired sensitivity to pain; paralysis; malnutrition; impaired circulation; incontinence; obesity; edema; anemia; confusion; and warm, moist skin areas.

8. The urine glucose level may be a poor indicator of blood glucose elevation in older adults because of their increased threshold for urinary glucose excretion.

9. Problems stemming from a high-fiber diet include the inclusion of more food than an older adult reasonably can consume; eating difficulties caused by poor tooth condition or ill-fitting dentures; and such GI disturbances as flatulence, distention, and diarrhea.

10. The most common fracture sites in older adults are the vertebrae, upper end of the femur (hip fracture), distal end of the radius (Colles' fracture), and proximal end of the humerus.

11. The nursing goal for older adults with glaucoma is to prevent vision loss.

12. Age-related changes contributing to hypertension in older adults include (any three) aortic rigidity, reduced baroreceptor sensitivity, decreased arteriolar lumen size, reduced glomerular filtration rate, changes in the renin-angiotensin system, and hormonal and cardiovascular changes.

13. Hypothyroidism sometimes is hard to detect in older adults because its signs and symptoms may resemble normal aging changes.

14. In older adults, myocardial infarction may cause such complications as (any three) serious arrhythmias, CHF, cardiogenic shock, digitalis toxicity, and cardiac rupture.

15. Heberden nodes develop in distal interphalangeal finger joints.

16. Common fracture sites in older adults with osteoporosis are the wrist (Colles' fracture), vertebrae (T_{12} and L_1), and hip.

17. The leading causes of renal impairment in older adults are urinary tract infection and renovascular disease secondary to hypertension.

18. In older adults, weight loss and CHF may be the predominant signs of thyrotoxicosis.

19. Conditions predisposing older adults to urinary stasis, retention, and obstruction include urethral or ureteral stenosis or strictures, renal calculi, immobility, tumors, neurologic changes caused by cerebrovascular accident (CVA), cystocele (in women), and prostatic hypertrophy (in men).

20. Deep-vein thrombosis involves calf veins, including the peroneal and posterior tibial veins.

CHAPTER 6

1. Two types of functional assessment that the nurse can conduct on older adults are assessment of activities of daily living (ADLs) and assessment of instrumental ADLs.

2. In a patient with sensory deprivation, the nurse should expect such cognitive function changes as confusion, disorientation, general slowing of intellectual activity, difficulty with concentration and abstract thinking, impaired problem solving, and inability to think coherently.

3. When caring for a patient with impaired hearing, the nurse can use such techniques as facing the patient, getting the patient's attention through touch or eye contact, sitting or standing so that the patient can see the nurse's lips, speaking slowly and distinctly, speaking in a voice loud enough to be heard without shouting, using short phrases, using appropriate body language, eliminating as much background noise as possible, and using a speaking tube or hearing horn (if the patient has a severe hearing impairment).

4. The patient with poor visual accommodation typically holds objects at a distance to focus on them properly.

5. The sense of smell begins to decline at about age 45.

6. Aging causes decreased skin turgor.

7. Conditions that commonly limit mobility in older adults include paresthesia, arthritis, neuromotor disturbances, fractures, energy-depleting illness, CVA, joint or foot pain, angina, and peripheral vascular disease.

8. Four types of urinary incontinence are stress incontinence, overflow incontinence, neurogenic incontinence, and urgency incontinence.

CHAPTER 7

1. Physical factors contributing to falls in older adults include (any two) muscle weakness, gait changes, decreased sensory awareness, and visual impairment.

2. To monitor temperature in an older adult with hypothermia, the nurse should take the patient's temperature rectally.

3. Heat exhaustion is less severe than heat stroke and is characterized by orthostatic hypotension, malaise, irritability, anxiety, tachypnea, tachycardia, moderate temperature increase, headache, dizziness, and syncope. Heat stroke is characterized by severe tachycardia, severe tachypnea, severe frank hypotension, alteration in consciousness, and a rectal temperature above 105° F (40.5° C).

4. In an older adult with high-altitude cerebral edema, the nurse should expect increasingly severe headaches, confusion, emotional lability, hallucinations, ataxia, and weakness.

5. Factors that predispose an older adult to fires and burns include (any two) a decreased sense of smell, overloading of old circuitry, lack of visual acuity to detect frayed electrical cords, and decreased sensitivity to heat and pain.

6. Drug absorption, distribution, metabolism, and excretion are altered in older adults.

7. The nurse should advise older adults to avoid isometric exercises because these exercises stimulate the vagovagal response and raise blood pressure.

8. Depression is the most common cause of sleep disturbance in older adults.

9. During phase 1, exhilaration occurs, followed by a letdown; during phase 2, the retiree experiments with new activities; during phase 3, the retiree becomes disenchanted; and during phase 4, new patterns emerge.

10. The best predictors of sexual behavior in older adults are past sexual activity and enjoyment.

11. When performing oral care, the nurse should moisten and clean the patient's mouth with normal saline solution and avoid using solutions containing alcohol.

12. Nutritional deficiencies in older adults usually result from inappropriate food selection rather than inadequate food intake.

13. Common problems in hospitalized older adults include (any three) poor eating habits, urinary incontinence, fecal incontinence, constipation, insomnia, confusion, and pain.

CHAPTER 8

1. Causes of caregiver stress include multiple demands, isolation, loneliness, and low morale.

2. Lack of transportation may cause social withdrawal, poor nutrition, lack of medical care, and loss of independence.

3. The focus of acute care is on curing and healing.

4. Long-term care (LTC) skilled-nursing facilities provide care for patients who are chronically ill or disabled and need full-day nursing care. LTC intermediate-care facilities provide custodial care and personal-care services for patients requiring nursing care less than 24 hours a day.

CHAPTER 9

1. Behavioral findings that suggest abuse in an older adult include (any three) excessive fear; compliant or dependent behavior; self-blame; avoidance of the abuser's touch; expression of concern that the abuser is taking the person's money or property; lack of needed supervision; lack of money, transportation, or other support; and inappropriate home maintenance.

2. A conservatorship is an arrangement whereby a person or institution is designated to take over and protect the interests of a person judged to be incompetent.

3. To give valid consent, a person must be competent and informed fully of all risks and benefits of a procedure or treatment.

4. Appropriate nursing actions to take when a patient decides not to prolong life by extraordinary means include supporting the patient and family in decision making, supporting nurses and physicians who implement right-to-die policies, and ensuring that supportive care is maintained.

CHAPTER 10

1. Factors contributing to problems in financing social welfare programs include (any two) changes in economic conditions, higher unemployment rates, rapid inflation, and lower productivity.

2. The Amendment to Age Discrimination in Employment Act (1978) raised the mandatory retirement age to 70.

3. Eligibility for welfare programs is based on economic status.

4. Hospital expenses account for 42% of the health care costs of older adults.

5. Medicare part A covers inpatient hospital care, medically necessary inpatient care in a skilled nursing facility after a hospital stay, home health care, and hospice care.

6. Types of private health insurance available to older adults include (any three) Medicare supplementary programs, catastrophic or major medical expense coverage, health maintenance organization insurance, employer group insurance, and association group insurance.

7. To help older adults deal with the economic aspects of health care, the nurse can recognize the cost constraints of older adults' income restrictions,

plan care to contain costs, become familiar with current Medicare and Medicaid requirements and limitations, become familiar with community resources, provide information and direction to help older adults contact appropriate agencies, and caution older adults considering Medicare supplementation to investigate these programs thoroughly.

CHAPTER 11

1. Roles for the gerontologic nurse include (any three) communicator, planner, case finder, caregiver, comforter, teacher, rehabilitator, and coordinator.

2. Gerontologic nursing represents care and treatment of older adults from a holistic standpoint, not just as diseased or sick persons. Geriatric nursing focuses on care of sick persons.

3. Requirements for certification as a gerontologic nurse practitioner include successful completion of the certification examination, a master's degree, and practice experience.

4. Gerontologic nursing functions in community care include (any three) identifying the patient's health, social, or economic needs; providing referrals to the appropriate professional or agency; explaining diagnosis and treatment to the patient and family; evaluating the patient's compliance with and response to treatment; using clinic and home visits for health promotion; teaching and advising the patient and family; evaluating the patient's ability to live independently; acting as an advocate for older adults; and encouraging older adults to become advocates on their own behalf.

5. Issues affecting the gerontologic nursing role include (any two) gerontologic nursing research, advocacy, changes in health care delivery, development of ANA councils to set standards, movement of practitioner education into graduate nursing programs, efforts to obtain third-party payment for nurse practitioners, and demonstration projects.

C: Resources

National organizations on aging and age-related health problems are listed below. Consult a telephone directory for state and local agencies.

Government agencies on aging

Administration on Aging
Department of Health and Human
  Services
330 Independence Ave. S.W.
Washington, DC 20201

Architectural and Transportation
  Barriers
Compliance Board
330 C St. S.W., Room 1010
Washington, DC 20202

National Institute on Aging
Building 31C
9000 Rockville Pike
Bethesda, MD 20205

Health organizations on aging

American Association for Geriatric
  Psychiatry
P.O. Box 376-A
Greenbelt, MD 20770

American Geriatrics Society
770 Lexington Ave., Suite 400
New York, NY 10021

American Health Care Association
  (nursing homes)
1201 L St. N.W.
Washington, DC 20005

American Nurses' Association
Council on Gerontological Nursing
2420 Pershing Rd.
Kansas City, MO 64108

American Society for Geriatric
  Dentistry
211 E. Chicago Ave.
Chicago, IL 60611

Gerontological Society of America
1275 K St. N.W., Suite 350
Washington, DC 20005

National Association for Home Care
519 C St. N.E.
Washington, DC 20002

National Hospice Organization
1901 N. Moore St., Suite 901
Arlington, VA 22209

Social welfare organizations on aging

American Association of Retired
  Persons
1909 K St. N.W.
Washington, DC 20049

Gray Panthers
311 S. Juniper St., Suite 601
Philadelphia, PA 19107

Institute for Retired Professionals
New School for Social Research
66 W. 12th St.
New York, NY 10011

National Center on Black Aging
1424 K St. N.W., Suite 500
Washington, DC 20005

National Council on the Aging
600 Maryland Ave. S.W., Suite 100 W
Washington, DC 20024

National Institute on Adult Daycare
c/o National Council on the Aging
600 Maryland Ave. S.W., Suite 100 W
Washington, DC 20024

National Senior Citizens Law Center
1052 W. Sixth St., Suite 700
Los Angeles, CA 90017

Other health and social welfare organizations for older adults

Alcoholism

Alcoholics Anonymous World Services
P.O. Box 459, Grand Central Station
New York, NY 10163

Al-Anon Family Group Headquarters
1372 Broadway
New York, NY 10018

Arthritis

Arthritis Foundation
1314 Spring St. N.W.
Atlanta, GA 30309

Cancer

American Cancer Society
1599 Clifton Rd. NE
Atlanta, GA 30329-4251

Heart disease

American Heart Association
7320 Greenville Ave.
Dallas, TX 75231

Impaired hearing

Alexander Graham Bell Association for the Deaf
3417 Volta Pl. N.W.
Washington, DC 20007

National Association of the Deaf
814 Thayer Ave.
Silver Spring, MD 20910

National Hearing Aid Society
20361 Middlebelt Rd.
Livonia, MI 48152

Kidney disorders

National Kidney Foundation
30 E. 33rd St., 11th Floor
New York, NY 10016

Mental health disorders

National Mental Health Association
1021 Prince St.
Alexandria, VA 22314

Respiratory disorders

American Lung Association
1740 Broadway
New York, NY 10019

Speech problems

American Speech-Language-Hearing Association
10801 Rockville Pike
Rockville, MD 20852

Stroke

Stroke Club International
805 12th St.
Galveston, TX 77550

Impaired vision

American Council of the Blind
1010 Vermont Ave. N.W., Suite 1100
Washington, DC 20005

American Foundation for the Blind
15 W. 16th St.
New York, NY 10011

American Printing House for the Blind
P.O. Box 6085
1839 Frankfort Ave.
Louisville, KY 40206

Blinded Veterans Association
477 H St. N.W., Suite 800
Washington, DC 20001

National Society to Prevent Blindness
500 E. Remington Rd.
Schaumburg, IL 60173

Selected References

American Nurses' Association. *Gerontological Nurses in Clinical Settings: Survey Analysis.* Kansas City, Mo.: American Nurses' Association, 1986.

American Nurses' Association. *Gerontological Nursing Curriculum: Survey Analysis and Recommendations.* Kansas City, Mo.: American Nurses' Association, 1986.

Birren J.E., and Schaie, K.W., eds. *Handbook of the Psychology of Aging,* 3rd ed. New York: Van Nostrand Reinhold Co., 1990.

Carnevali, D.L., and Patrick, M. *Nursing Management for the Elderly,* 2nd ed. Philadelphia: J.B. Lippincott Co., 1986.

Dychtwald, K. *Wellness and Health Promotion for the Elderly.* Rockville, Md.: Aspen Systems Corp., 1986.

Ebersole, P., and Hess, P. *Toward Health Aging: Human Needs and Nursing Response,* 3rd ed. St. Louis: Mosby-Year Book, Inc., 1990.

Eliopoulis, C., ed. *Health Assessment of the Older Adult.* 2nd ed. Menlo Park, Calif.: Addison-Wesley Publishing Co., 1990.

Foreman, M.D. "Acute Confusional States in the Elderly: An Algorithm," *Dimensions of Critical Care Nursing* 3(4): 207-15, 1984.

A Profile of Older Americans: 1990. Washington, D.C.: Program Resources Department, American Association of Retired Persons in cooperation with the Administration on Aging, 1991.

Hart, G. "Strokes Causing Left vs. Right Hemiplegia: Different Effects and Nursing Implications," *Geriatric Nursing* 1(1): 39-43, January/February 1983.

Mace, N.L., and Rabins, R.U. *The 36-Hour Day.* New York: Hopkins, 1991.

Matteson, M.A., and McConnell, E.S. *Gerontological Nursing Concepts and Practice.* Philadelphia: W.B. Saunders, 1988.

National League for Nursing. *Overcoming the Bias of Ageism in Long Term Care.* New York: National League for Nursing, 1985.

Oppeneer, J.E., and Vervoren, T.M. *Gerontological Pharmacology: A Resource for Health Practitioners.* St. Louis: C.V. Mosby Co., 1983.

Rossman, I. *Clinical Geriatrics.* Philadelphia: J.B. Lippincott Co., 1986.

Simonson, W. *Medications and the Elderly: A Guide for Promoting Proper Use.* Rockville, Md.: Aspen Systems Corp., 1984.

Steffl, B.M., ed. *Handbook of Gerontological Nursing.* New York: Von Nostrand Reinhold Co., 1984.

Yurich, A.V.G., et al. *The Aged Person and the Nursing Process,* 3rd ed. East Norwalk, Conn.: Appleton-Century-Crofts, 1989.

Index

i refers to an illustration; t, to a table.

Notes

Notes

Notes

Notes